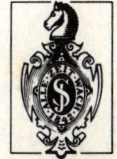

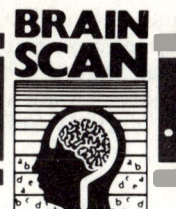
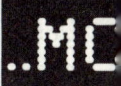

**BRAIN SCAN**

MCQ≡....MCQ≡....MCQ≡... ..MC

Gordon S. Laing

# Accident and Emergency Medicine

Springer-Verlag
London Berlin Heidelberg New York
Paris Tokyo

Gordon S. Laing, FRCS
Consultant in Accident and Emergency Medicine, Hope
Hospital, Salford, Honorary Associate Lecturer in Surgery,
University of Manchester, and Chairman, Specialty Training
Group, North West Region

Publisher's note: the "Brainscan" logo is reproduced by courtesy of The
Editor, *Geriatric Medicine*, Modern Medicine GB Ltd.

ISBN 3–540–19508–4 Springer-Verlag Berlin Heidelberg New York
ISBN 0–387–19508–4 Springer-Verlag New York Berlin Heidelberg

British Library Cataloguing in Publication Data
Laing, Gordon S. (Gordon Stewart) 1924–
    Accident and emergency medicine
    1. Medicine. Emergency treatment.
    I. Title
616'.025.
ISBN 3–540–19508–4

Library of Congress Cataloging-in-Publication Data
Laing, Gordon S., 1924–
Accident and emergency medicine.
(Brainscan MCQ's)
1. Emergency medicine–Examinations, questions, etc. I. Title. II. Series.
[DNLM: 1. Accidents–examination questions. 2. Emergency Medicine–
examination questions. WB 18 L187a] RC86.9.L35 1988    616'.025'076
87–37682
ISBN 0–387–19508–4

Phototypesetting by Tradeset Photosetting, 10 Garden Court Business
Centre, Tewin Road, Welwyn Garden City, Hertfordshire, AL7 1BH.
Printed by The Bath Press, Lower Bristol Road, Bath, Avon.

2128/3916-543210

Dedicated to three A's
Ann, Alexandra and Adam

# Preface

This little book has been written primarily for the senior house officer in Accident and Emergency and the registrar pursuing a career in the specialty. I hope also that it will be of interest to medical students. Thanks to the initiative of Professor Miles Irving, Professor of Surgery, University of Manchester, medical students have been taught Accident and Emergency in Hope Hospital since 1974. Many of the answers to the questions here have been elaborated as a result of their enquiring minds. It has been a pleasure to teach them.

MCQs should be informative and entertaining and not regarded as a tiresome chore merely because of self-assessment scoring. I have omitted the boxes and the "don't know" response. The answers are either true or false. I have attempted to slot the questions into various sections with some degree of sequence, but there is an inevitable overlap particularly with regard to the sections on the unresponsive patient, poisoning and injury. The final section is a selected mixture of Accident and Emergency and I thought "Pot-pourri" an appropriate title. I have enjoyed compiling the questions and I hope that both undergraduates and postgraduates will find reading them a painless and worthwhile exercise.

Finally my thanks are due to my secretary Eileen Bates for her typing and patience.

Salford                                          Gordon S. Laing

# Contents

# 1. *The Unresponsive Patient*

**Q.1.1**   **In managing an unresponsive patient you immediately:**

   a. Listen to the heart
   b. Examine the central nervous system
   c. Feel the carotid pulses
   d. Examine the airway
   e. Ascertain whether breathing

**Q.1.2**   **Cardiac arrest is due to:**

   a. Ventricular fibrillation
   b. Ventricular asystole
   c. Atrial fibrillation
   d. Electromechanical dissociation
   e. Complete heart block

**For answers see over**

# Answers

**A.1.1**  a. F
          b. F
          c. T
          d. T
          e. T

**A.1.2**  a. T
          b. T
          c. F
          d. T
          e. F

Defibrillation has greatly increased survival in cardiac arrest due to ventricular fibrillation resulting from acute myocardial infarction. A high mortality persists in ventricular asystole and electromechanical dissociation.

Ventricular asystole results from acute myocardial infarction, hypoxia, hypovolaemia and from defibrillation.

Electromechanical dissociation (EMD) is continued electrical activity without pump action. It is due to acute myocardial infarction, acute cardiac tamponade, massive pulmonary embolism, tension pneumothorax, hyperkalaemia and hypoglycaemia.

**Q.1.3** **In the management of ventricular asystole the first-line drug is:**

    a. Adrenaline
    b. Atropine
    c. Calcium
    d. Isoprenaline
    e. Sodium bicarbonate

**For answers see over**

# *Answers*

**A.1.3**  a. F
       b. T
       c. F
       d. F
       e. F

It is likely that in ventricular asystole the heart is rendered immobile by excessive vagal parasympathetic activity due to receptor stimulation. Atropine can abolish this parasympathetic drive.

In ventricular asystole the endogenous catecholamine levels are very high, particularly if preceded by acute myocardial infarction. The levels are well above those reported to exert physiological and pharmacological effects on the myocardium and may be as high as 300 nmol/l. A plasma level of 0.5 nmol/l will increase the heart rate. There would seem to be little point in administering further exogenous catecholamine in an attempt to stimulate the arrested myocardium. When the parasympathetic activity is removed the heart may then be able to respond to this high level of endogenous catecholamine.

Calcium is of little value in cardiac arrest. It increases cardiac muscle spasticity and oxygen requirement and causes cellular death. If given to a digitalised patient there is danger of severe dysrhythmias. It is better reserved for hyperkalaemia and hypocalcaemia. Calcium antagonists are preferable and may preserve the myocardium around the infarction zone. Cardiac contractility is depressed with a consequent reduction in myocardial oxygen demand.

Isoprenaline is a beta-adrenergic drug which can increase cardiac output but is toxic and can induce ventricular fibrillation. It increases myocardial oxygen consumption and causes myocardial cell necrosis. It is contraindicated in cardiac arrest.

Sodium bicarbonate should be used only in the unwitnessed arrest – that is an arrest of unknown duration with prolonged hypoxia – and then given as a maximum of 50 ml of 8.4% solution into the central vein. The acid–base state should be assessed by analysis of an arterial blood sample. It should not be given immediately in a witnessed arrest because there is a metabolic acidosis and the fall in pH shifts the oxygen dissociation curve to the right, allowing oxygen to drain from the stagnant circulation into the tissues. If the sodium bicarbonate is given early in cardiopulmonary resuscitation it will prevent this shift of the oxygen dissociation curve and reduce the chance of survival.

**Q.1.4** **Atropine in ventricular asystole is administered:**

    a. Via a peripheral vein
    b. Via a central vein
    c. Via a cut down vein in the ankle
    d. Directly into the heart
    e. Down the endotracheal tube

**Q.1.5** **In "new" cardiopulmonary resuscitation:**

    a. The common carotid artery blood flow is increased
    b. The systemic arterial systolic pressure is raised
    c. The diastolic pressure is raised
    d. Cerebral perfusion is improved
    e. Myocardial perfusion is improved

**For answers see over**

# Answers

**A.1.4**   a. F
               b. T
               c. F
               d. T
               e. T

Atropine should be given in a bolus of 2 mg directly into the heart subxiphisternally or via the central vein.

There is no point in using a peripheral vein when there is no circulation.

Endotracheal administration is less effective.

**A.1.5**   a. T
               b. T
               c. F
               d. F
               e. F

The increase in common carotid flow demonstrated in animal experiments is directed towards the external rather than the internal carotid artery.

There is a slight increase in systolic blood pressure.

The diastolic pressure falls.

The rise in intrathoracic pressure may cause increased intracranial pressure thus impairing cerebral perfusion.

The coronary arteries fill during diastole and as the diastolic pressure falls myocardial perfusion is reduced.

*Note:*

"New" cardiopulmonary resuscitation is simultaneous closed chest cardiac compression with ventilation, at a rate of 40 per minute with 60% compression duration and airway pressures of 60–110 cmH$_2$O.

**Q.1.6** **Cardiogenic shock occurs in:**

a. Acute myocardial infarction
b. Cardiac tamponade
c. Massive pulmonary embolism
d. Cardiac contusion
e. Ventricular, septal or valve rupture

For answers see over

# Answers

**A.1.6**   a. T
         b. T
         c. T
         d. T
         e. T

**Fundamentals of Cardiac Life Support**

<u>A</u>irway
<u>B</u>reathing
<u>C</u>irculation
<u>D</u>efibrillation

**Witnessed Collapse**

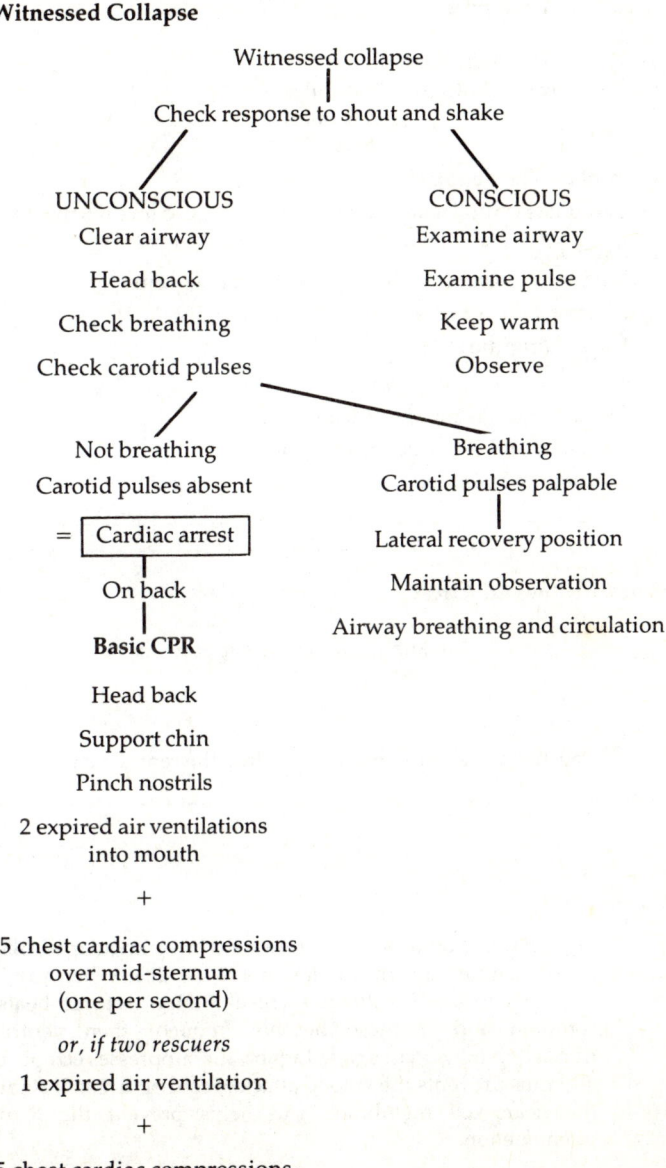

Witnessed collapse
|
Check response to shout and shake

**UNCONSCIOUS**

Clear airway

Head back

Check breathing

Check carotid pulses

Not breathing
Carotid pulses absent

= | Cardiac arrest |
|
On back
|
**Basic CPR**

Head back

Support chin

Pinch nostrils

2 expired air ventilations
into mouth

+

15 chest cardiac compressions
over mid-sternum
(one per second)

*or, if two rescuers*

1 expired air ventilation

+

5 chest cardiac compressions

**CONSCIOUS**

Examine airway

Examine pulse

Keep warm

Observe

Breathing
Carotid pulses palpable

Lateral recovery position

Maintain observation

Airway breathing and circulation

**Advanced Cardiopulmonary Resuscitation (CPR) or Advanced Cardiac Life Support**

1. *Ventricular fibrillation*
   Defibrillate ×3 rapidly   200 joules
                                          300 joules
                                          300 joules
   Intubate and ventilate
   Cannulate central vein and give bolus of lignocaine 100 mg 2%

2. *Asystole*
   Intracardiac atropine 2 mg or into subclavian vein
   Intubate and ventilate
   Repeat atropine

3. *Electromechanical dissociation*
   Examine neck veins and feel the trachea
   Consider 5 ml 10% calcium chloride
   Intubate and ventilate

---

**The Unwitnessed Arrest**

Advanced cardiac life support

+

50 ml 8.4% sodium bicarbonate into the central vein

---

Lignocaine should be given routinely in ventricular fibrillation in the central vein in a bolus of 100 mg 2%. When the heart responds to cardiopulmonary resuscitation, ectopic beats are common and if these become frequent then ventricular fibrillation may occur again. Lignocaine suppresses ectopic beats and thus prevents the second attack of cardiac arrest. It stabilises the heart cell membrane and helps prevent the R on T phenomenon.

**Q.1.7**   **The commonest presentations of coma in an Accident and Emergency Department are:**

a. Head injury
b. Cerebrovascular lesion
c. Alcohol intoxication
d. Overdose
e. Hypoglycaemia

**Q.1.8**   **The following causes of unresponsiveness may be considered reversible:**

a. Heroin toxicity
b. Mid-brain haemorrhage
c. Hypoglycaemia
d. Alcohol toxicity
e. Adams–Stokes attack

For answers see over

# Answers

**A.1.7**   a.  T
           b.  T
           c.  T
           d.  T
           e.  T

The term coma is from the Greek word meaning deep sleep and is often used to describe a prolonged state of unconsciousness. Unresponsiveness is probably a better term.

**A.1.8**   a.  T
           b.  F
           c.  T
           d.  T
           e.  T

In heroin toxicity give naloxone intravenously commencing with 0.8 mg.

Mid-brain haemorrhage is irreversible.

Hypoglycaemia is usually due to insulin overdosage and responds dramatically to 50 ml 50% dextrose IV.

Alcohol toxicity may be reversed with 200 ml 20% laevulose IV.

A patient with an Adams–Stokes drop attack due to bradycardia and cerebral ischaemia usually regains consciousness but should be referred for a pacemaker.

**Q.1.9** Dilated fixed pupils in an unresponsive patient occur in:

    a. Heroin toxicity
    b. Cardiac arrest
    c. Death
    d. Amphetamine toxicity
    e. Alcohol intoxication

**Q.1.10** Overdose with the following drugs causes dilatation of the pupils in the absence of hypoxic brain damage:

    a. Barbiturates
    b. Hyoscine
    c. Tricyclics
    d. Glutethimide
    e. Lomotil

**For answers see over**

# Answers

**A.1.9**    a.  F
           b.  T
           c.  T
           d.  T
           e.  T

The pupils are constricted in heroin toxicity.

In cardiac arrest the pupils are dilated and there is no reaction to light. Examine the optic fundi. If the retinal vessels are engorged with blood continue resuscitation.

In death the pupils are dilated and fixed to light. Examine the optic fundi to confirm death. "Cattle trucking" is seen in the retinal vessels, which then drain and the optic fundi become white.

Amphetamines dilate the pupils by sympathomimetic action but there may be a light reflex.

Alcohol dilates the pupils but the light reflex may be retained. If the patient has been found lying in the street, X-ray the skull.

**A.1.10**    a.  F
           b.  T
           c.  T
           d.  T
           e.  T

Pupillary reaction is variable in barbiturate toxicity. Hippus may occur, alternating dilation and constriction.

Tricyclic antidepressant drugs inhibit pupillary constriction by their anticholinergic action.

Glutethimide has an atropine-like action.

Lomotil contains atropine.

**Q.1.11** **Pin-point pupils in an unresponsive patient are due to:**

a. Diabetic ketosis
b. Pontine haemorrhage
c. Opiate toxicity
d. Salicylate poisoning
e. Paracetamol poisoning

**Q.1.12** **An ipsilateral dilated fixed pupil in an unresponsive patient may be due to:**

a. Extradural haemorrhage
b. Hypoglycaemia
c. Horner syndrome
d. Subarachnoid haemorrhage
e. Aneurysm of the circle of Willis

**For answers see over**

# Answers

**A.1.11**  a.  F
           b.  T
           c.  T
           d.  F
           e.  F

Note the pyrexia in pontine haemorrhage.

**A.1.12**  a.  T
           b.  F
           c.  F
           d.  T
           e.  T

The dilatation of the pupil in extradural haemorrhage is due to compression of the oculomotor nerve from herniation of the hippocampal gyrus over the free edge of the tentorium.

Pupils are equal in hypoglycaemia and may be dilated.

Horner syndrome is characterised by a constricted pupil due to sympathetic nerve paralysis or injury.

In subarachnoid haemorrhage due to a ruptured aneurysm of the posterior cerebral artery, the superior cerebellar artery or the posterior communicating artery, the oculomotor nerve will be involved.

The oculomotor nerve passes between the posterior cerebral and superior cerebellar arteries before entering the cavernous sinus. The aneurysm may compress the oculomotor nerve prior to rupture producing a dilated pupil.

**Q.1.13** **In an unresponsive patient with a temperature below 35 °C the diagnosis is:**

a. Hypoglycaemia
b. Hypothermia
c. Myxoedema
d. Overdose
e. Alcohol intoxication

**For answers see over**

**A.1.13**  a.  F
      b.  T
      c.  T
      d.  T
      e.  T

The temperature is normal in hypoglycaemia unless the patient has been found in a cold environment.

The patient will have been exposed to a cold environment. Consider drugs in the elderly – chlorpromazine particularly lowers body temperature. The patient may have an illness or injury – cerebrovascular catastrophe or a fractured neck of femur may be the reason an elderly person has not been able to get up. Acute hypothermia is usually due to immersion in cold water.

Myxoedema and hypothermia may be associated but it is not a common presentation in an Accident and Emergency Department.

In the late stages of self-poisoning the temperature falls.

Alcohol causes vasodilatation and this results in a fall in body temperature.

**Q.1.14** **In an unresponsive patient a temperature over 38 °C can be due to:**

a. Cerebrovascular lesion
b. Infection
c. Head injury
d. Hypovolaemia
e. Epilepsy

**Q.1.15** **In an unresponsive patient with a head injury bleeding from the ears is a sign of:**

a. Raised intracranial pressure
b. Fractured parietal bone
c. Subdural haematoma
d. Extradural haemorrhage
e. Fractured base of skull

**For answers see over**

# Answers

**A.1.14**  a.  T
           b.  T
           c.  F
           d.  F
           e.  F

In mid-brain haemorrhage, usually pontine haemorrhage, the temperature is over 39 °C. The pupils are pin-point.

The temperature is high in meningitis and encephalitis. Remember infectious diseases may cause febrile convulsions in children. In cerebral malaria the temperature can be over 40 °C. It is always wise to examine slides for malaria parasites if the diagnosis is in doubt.

In head injury the temperature is not usually raised but the blood pressure often is.

The temperature in hypovolaemia is usually normal unless the patient has bled in a cold environment.

In epilepsy the temperature is normal.

**A.1.15**  a.  F
           b.  F
           c.  F
           d.  F
           e.  T

Bleeding from the ears is usually blood-stained cerebrospinal fluid and is due to fracture of the middle cranial fossa. It feels watery when rubbed between finger and thumb.

**Q.1.16  Criteria for skull X-ray after head injury are:**

a. Loss of consciousness and/or amnesia
b. Neurological signs
c. Cerebrospinal fluid from ear or nose
d. Suspected penetrating injury
e. Alcohol intoxication

**Q.1.17  Criteria for admission following head injury are:**

a. Confusion or depression of level of consciousness
b. Skull fracture
c. Neurological signs, significant headache and persistent vomiting
d. Difficulty in assessing patient following alcohol intoxication or epilepsy
e. Patient's social conditions, e.g. lack of responsible adult/ relative

**For answers see over**

# Answers

**A.1.16**  a. T
        b. T
        c. T
        d. T
        e. T

**A.1.17**  a. T
        b. T
        c. T
        d. T
        e. T

**Glasgow Coma Scale**

| EYES | Open | Spontaneously | 4 |
|---|---|---|---|
| | | To verbal command | 3 |
| | | To pain | 2 |
| | No response | | 1 |
| BEST MOTOR RESPONSE | To verbal command | Obeys | 6 |
| | To painful stimulus | Localises pain | 5 |
| | | Flexion – withdrawal | 4 |
| | | Flexion – abnormal | 3 |
| | | Extension | 2 |
| | | No response | 1 |
| BEST VERBAL RESPONSE | | Oriented and converses | 5 |
| | | Disorientated and converses | 4 |
| | | Inappropriate words | 3 |
| | | Incomprehensible sounds | 3 |
| | | No response | 1 |
| TOTAL | | | 3–15 |

**Q.1.18**  **A white opacity seen on a skull X-ray may be due to:**
  a. Artefact
  b. Fracture of the skull
  c. Dressing
  d. Suture line
  e. Depressed fracture

**Q.1.19**  **Extradural haemorrhage:**
  a. May occur in rugby
  b. Is characterised by a lucid interval
  c. Has blood-stained cerebrospinal fluid
  d. Is frequently bilateral
  e. Has pupillary signs

**For answers see over**

# Answers

**A.1.18**   a. T
          b. F
          c. T
          d. F
          e. T

A fracture of the skull is seen as a black line.

The edge of a dressing can usually be identified.

Suture lines are black.

A depressed fracture is white and usually crescent-shaped.

**A.1.19**   a. T
          b. T
          c. F
          d. F
          e. T

Often the patient is a young male with a history of loss of consciousness after head injury playing rugby which may be followed by a lucid interval. The lucid interval occurs in 20%–25% cases.

The cerebrospinal fluid is clear.

Extradural haemorrhage is rarely bilateral.

The diagnosis is confirmed by CT scan.

The consensual reaction should be included in the examination of the dilated pupil. In extradural haemorrhage the pupil on the side of the bleed is often dilated and fixed to light, but the other pupil reacts consensually. If the light is shone into the other pupil, that pupil constricts but there is no consensual constriction of the dilated pupil. This is because of interruption of the efferent pathway of the light reflex involving the oculomotor nerve.

An extradural haemorrhage has an Abbreviated Injury Scale (AIS) of:
    4 if < 100 ml
    5 if > 100 ml

A subdural haematoma is similarly scored.

**Q.1.20  In subarachnoid haemorrhage:**

    a.  The aneurysms are due to syphilis
    b.  The aneurysms are multiple in over 20% of cases
    c.  The aneurysms are due to atherosclerosis
    d.  Berry aneurysms of the circle of Willis are usually responsible
    e.  The affected are usually elderly

**Q.1.21  An anterior cranial fossa fracture may present with:**

    a.  Proptosis
    b.  Bleeding with cerebrospinal fluid from the ears
    c.  Bruising of the orbits
    d.  Aerocoele formation
    e.  Papilloedema

**Q.1.22  Indications for urgent referral to a neurosurgeon are:**

    a.  Deteriorating consciousness
    b.  Developing focal signs
    c.  Dilating pupils
    d.  Bradycardia and/or rising blood pressure
    e.  Depressed fracture

**Q.1.23  The antibiotic of choice in middle cranial fossa fracture with otorrhoea is:**

    a.  Amoxicillin
    b.  Flucloxacillin
    c.  Penicillin
    d.  Tetracycline
    e.  Co-trimoxazole

**For answers see over**

# Answers

**A.1.20**  a. F
        b. T
        c. F
        d. T
        e. F

Subarachnoid haemorrhage affects the young and middle-aged.
It may occur in pregnancy and labour.

**A.1.21**  a. T
        b. F
        c. T
        d. T
        e. F

Panda eyes or racoon eyes are commonly seen in anterior cranial
fossa fracture.

**A.1.22**  a. T
        b. T
        c. T
        d. T
        e. T

**A.1.23**  a. F
        b. T
        c. F
        d. F
        e. F

**Q.1.24**   **An extensor plantar response may be elicited in:**

    a. Cerebral haemorrhage
    b. Hypoglycaemic coma
    c. Myxoedema
    d. Infants
    e. Hepatic coma

**Q.1.25**   **Diabetic coma:**

    a. Is due to infection, failure to take insulin and dietary indiscretion
    b. Is characterised by dehydration
    c. Is of sudden onset
    d. May be preceded by epigastric pain and vomiting
    e. Is characterised by air hunger

**For answers see over**

# Answers

**A.1.24**  a.  T
         b.  T
         c.  F
         d.  T
         e.  F

Hypoglycaemic coma may be confused with an upper motor neurone lesion. In the presence of sweating a blood sugar test should be done, particularly if there is a history of irritability and drunken behaviour prior to the unconsciousness. It is wise to do a blood sugar test on any patient who resists examination.

In myxoedema the reflexes are sluggish and the plantar responses flexor.

An extensor response is a normal physiological finding in young infants.

In hepatic coma the plantar response is flexor.

**A.1.25**  a.  T
         b.  T
         c.  F
         d.  T
         e.  T

**Q.1.26** **Hepatic coma due to cirrhosis:**

    a. May be preceded by haematemesis
    b. May be preceded by flapping tremor
    c. May be precipitated by diuretics
    d. May be precipitated by sedatives
    e. May be precipitated by a low-protein diet

**For answers see over**

# Answers

**A.1.26**  a.  T
         b.  T
         c.  T
         d.  T
         e.  F

---

**The Unresponsive or Comatose Patient**

**C**    Cardiac arrest
      Cardiac tamponade
      Cerebrovascular lesions
          Internal capsule haemorrhage
          Intraventricular haemorrhage
          Mid-brain haemorrhage
          Subarachnoid haemorrhage
          Basilar artery thrombosis
      Cerebral infarction with oedema
      Cerebral tumour
      Cerebral abscess
      Cerebral malaria
      Carbon dioxide retention

**O**    Overdose
      Opiates
      Other poisons

**M**   Metabolic
      Diabetes mellitus: diabetic ketosis, hypoglycaemia
      Hepatic: cirrhosis
      Uraemia: chronic nephritis

**A**    Alcohol intoxication
      Adams–Stokes attack
      Asphyxia
      Apnoea
      Aortic stenosis
      Anorexia nervosa
      Adult respiratory distress syndrome (ARDS)

*(Cont.)*

**The Unresponsive or Comatose Patient** (*Cont.*)

**T**    Trauma
        Head injury: extradural **haemorrhage, subdural** haematoma
        Cervical spine injury
        Chest injury
        Abdomen and pelvis injury
        Multiple injuries
    Terminal states: carcinomatosis

**O**    Ominous infections
        Encephalitis
        Meningitis
        Malaria
        Septicaemia
        Cholera
        AIDS

**S**    Shock
        Cardiogenic
        Hypovolaemic: blood, plasma, fluid loss
        Neurogenic
        Anaphylactic
    Suicide attempts: slashed throat, wrist
    Stab wounds
    Shotgun wounds
    Snake bite
    Spider bite
    Suprarenal haemorrhage
    Sunstroke
    Strangulation

**E**    Epilepsy
    Exposure
        Hypothermia
        Hyperthermia
    Embolism, massive pulmonary
    Encephalopathy
    Endocrine
        Hypopituitarism
        Addison's disease
        Hypothyroidism
    Ectopic pregnancy rupture
    Electrocution

# 2. Poisoning

**Q.2.1    Salicylate poisoning causes:**

    a.  Respiratory alkalosis
    b.  Metabolic acidosis
    c.  Loss of bicarbonate in the urine
    d.  Hyperkalaemia
    e.  Dehydration

**Q.2.2    The early stage of salicylate poisoning is characterised by:**

    a.  Epigastric pain
    b.  Vomiting
    c.  Sweating
    d.  Tinnitus
    e.  Subnormal temperature

**Q.2.3    Metabolic acidosis occurs as the result of:**

    a.  Loss of bicarbonate
    b.  Presence of salicylic acid in the blood
    c.  Inhibition of citric acid cycle enzymes
    d.  Increase of lactic and pyruvic acids
    e.  Ketosis

**For answers see over**

# Answers

**A.2.1**   a. T
           b. T
           c. T
           d. F
           e. T

Salicylates stimulate the respiratory centre producing a respiratory alkalosis.

There may be severe hypokalaemia.

**A.2.2**   a. T
           b. T
           c. T
           d. T
           e. F

There is hyperpyrexia.

**A.2.3**   a. T
           b. T
           c. T
           d. T
           e. T

The ketosis is produced by the stimulation of fat metabolism.

Protein catabolism is accelerated, producing an increase in circulating amino acids.

**Q.2.4**   **Blood salicylate levels of:**

    a.  100–300 mg/l indicate some toxicity
    b.  300–500 mg/l indicate mild toxicity
    c.  500–700 mg/l indicate moderate toxicity
    d.  700–1000 mg/l indicate severe toxicity
    e.  Over 1000 mg/l indicate very severe toxicity

**Q.2.5**   **The treatment of salicylate poisoning is by:**

    a.  Gastric lavage
    b.  Correction of dehydration
    c.  Correction of metabolic acidosis with IV bicarbonate
    d.  Vitamin K 10 mg IV
    e.  Forced alkaline diuresis if salicylate levels > 750 mg/l

**For answers see over**

# Answers

**A.2.4**   a.  T
            b.  T
            c.  T
            d.  T
            e.  T

**A.2.5**   a.  T
            b.  T
            c.  T
            d.  T
            e.  T

500 ml 5% dextrose plus 500 ml 1.2% sodium bicarbonate is given IV in the first hour. If urine output > 3 ml/min, repeat. Haemolysis is indicated if blood salicylate level > 100 mg/l.

---

**Syrup of Ipecacuanha Versus Gastric Lavage**

Syrup of ipecac is the method of choice for emptying the stomach in children and in conscious adults:

> 15 ml for children
> 30 ml for adults followed by 200 ml water and repeated after 20 minutes

Gastric lavage is indicated in the unconscious patient with an endotracheal tube in situ.
Gastric lavage should always be considered in salicylate poisoning and tricyclic antidepressant poisoning.

---

**Q.2.6    Distalgesic overdosage causes:**

    a.  Coma
    b.  Convulsions
    c.  Respiratory depression
    d.  Apnoea
    e.  Death

**Q.2.7    *N*–Acetylcysteine:**

    a.  Is effective in paracetamol poisoning
    b.  Is effective up to 20 hours after ingestion of paracetamol
    c.  Is effective up to 8 hours after ingestion of paracetamol
    d.  Restores depleted glutathione stores
    e.  Protects against hepatic failure

**Q.2.8    *Amanita phalloides* poisoning:**

    a.  Is toxic to liver and kidneys
    b.  May cause bloody vomiting
    c.  May be treated with benzylpenicillin
    d.  May be treated with sulphadimidine
    e.  Benzylpenicillin and sulphadimidine displace toxin from plasma and albumin and enhance urinary excretion

**For answers see over**

# Answers

**A.2.6**  a. T
  b. T
  c. T
  d. T
  e. T

Distalgesic is a combination of paracetamol 325 mg with dextropropoxyphene 32.5 mg, a narcotic analgesic. Overdosage is common and is potentiated by alcohol.

Treatment is by ventilation and IV naloxone and N-acetylcysteine.

**A.2.7**  a. T
  b. F
  c. T
  d. T
  e. T

The dose of N-acetylcysteine in paracetamol poisoning is 150 mg/kg in 200 ml 5% dextrose IV over 15 minutes followed by 50 mg/kg in 500 ml 5% dextrose over 4 hours.

Evacuation of the stomach by gastric lavage or syrup of ipecacuanha is indicated if the patient presents within 6 hours of ingestion of paracetamol.

Methionine may be given orally: 2.5 g initially, then 2.5 g 4-hourly for three doses to a total of 10 g over 12 hours.

Both N-acetylcysteine and methionine are effective and either should be administered within 8 hours of ingestion of paracetamol. Both act as glutathione precursors.

Paracetamol is available combined with methionine (Pameton: paracetamol 500 mg with methionine 250 mg) and is a safe analgesic.

**A.2.8**  a. T
  b. T
  c. T
  d. T
  e. T

**Q.2.9    Desferrioxamine:**

a. Is indicated in lead and mercury poisoning
b. Is indicated in iron poisoning
c. Acts by chelation of ferrous ions
d. May be used in the gastric lavage
e. May be given IV or IM

**Q.2.10   Overdosage with tricyclic antidepressants:**

a. Delay gastric emptying
b. Should be treated by gastric lavage within 12 hours of ingestion
c. Should be treated by activated charcoal following the lavage
d. Should be treated by forced diuresis
e. Should be treated by haemodialysis

**Q.2.11   Overdosage with non-steroidal anti-inflammatory drugs (NSAI):**

a. Gastric lavage should be performed if the patient presents within 4 hours of ingestion
b. Activated charcoal adsorbs propionic acid derivatives
c. Activated charcoal should be left in the stomach
d. Cimetidine 200 mg IV 6-hourly is advisable
e. Convulsions may be treated with diazepam 10 mg IV

**For answers see over**

# Answers

**A.2.9**  a.  F
b.  T
c.  T
d.  T
e.  T

2 g in 1 litre warm water should be used for the lavage and 5 g in 50 ml water left in the stomach.

2 g in 10 ml sterile water should be given IM, repeated after 12 hours. Alternatively 5 mg/kg per hour can be given slowly to a maximum of 80 mg/kg in 24 hours.

**A.2.10**  a.  T
b.  T
c.  T
d.  F
e.  F

**A.2.11**  a.  T
b.  T
c.  T
d.  T
e.  T

**Q.2.12    Corrosive poisoning should be treated by:**

a. Administration of syrup of ipecacuanha
b. Gastric lavage
c. An acid or an alkali
d. Administration of water
e. Administration of milk

**Q.2.13    Sodium calciumedetate:**

a. May be given for all metal poisons
b. Is indicated solely for lead poisoning
c. Acts by chelation of lead ions
d. Should be given with dimercaprol
e. Should be diluted with normal saline

**Q.2.14    Methylene blue:**

a. Is indicated in methaemoglobinaemia
b. Is indicated in phenol and cresol poisoning
c. Is indicated in cetrimide poisoning
d. Should be given with vitamin C
e. Should be administered rapidly

**Q.2.15    Fuller's Earth:**

a. Is indicated in paraquat poisoning
b. Is indicated if weedkiller splashed into the mouth
c. Acts by adsorption within the gut
d. Should be given with magnesium sulphate
e. Is given for 12 hours

**For answers see over**

# Answers

**A.2.12**  a. F
          b. F
          c. F
          d. T
          e. T

A patient who has swallowed a corrosive should be given water to dilute the corrosive. Vomiting should not be encouraged and gastric lavage never performed.

Alkalis should never be given for acid poisoning, nor acid for alkali poisoning. After dilution the gastric contents may be aspirated carefully through a nasogastric tube. Milk should be left in the stomach and the patient encouraged to swallow raw eggs.

**A.2.13**  a. F
          b. T
          c. T
          d. T
          e. T

75 mg/kg is given IV for 1 hour for 5 days.

**A.2.14**  a. T
          b. T
          c. T
          d. T
          e. F

2 mg/kg is given slowly IV.

200 mg vitamin C should be given three times daily for 3 days.

Methylene blue causes haemolysis in glucose-6-phosphate dehydrogenase deficiency.

**A.2.15**  a. T
          b. T
          c. T
          d. T
          e. F

250 ml of 30% suspension is given 4-hourly for 48 hours.

**Q.2.16 Dimercaprol:**
   a. Is indicated for arsenic poisoning
   b. Is indicated for copper poisoning
   c. May be given in lead poisoning
   d. Is contraindicated in mercury poisoning
   e. Acts by chelation of metal ions

**Q.2.17 Naloxone:**
   a. Is indicated in heroin toxicity
   b. Reverses severe respiratory depression in opiate toxicity
   c. Should be considered if the cause of unconsciousness is uncertain
   d. Causes improvement within minutes in opiate toxicity
   e. Acts as a competitive inhibitor at opiate receptor sites

**Q.2.18 Penicillamine:**
   a. Is indicated in zinc poisoning
   b. Is indicated in gold poisoning
   c. Is indicated in mercury and copper poisoning
   d. May be given in lead poisoning
   e. Acts by chelation of metal ions

**Q.2.19 Benztropine:**
   a. Is effective in all cases of dyskinesia
   b. Counteracts the extrapyramidal action of metoclopramide
   c. Counteracts the extrapyramidal action of phenothiazines
   d. Acts by competitive inhibition of muscarine receptors
   e. Blocks dopamine re-uptake

**For answers see over**

# Answers

**A.2.16** a. T
b. T
c. T
d. F
e. T

5 mg/kg is given IM 4-hourly for 2 days then 2.5 mg/kg twice daily for 2 days.

**A.2.17** a. T
b. T
c. T
d. T
e. T

Initial adult dose is 0.8 mg given IV, repeated. In children 0.005–0.01 mg/kg body weight should be given.

**A.2.18** a. T
b. T
c. T
d. T
e. T

250 mg – 2 g are given orally daily.

**A.2.19** a. F
b. T
c. T
d. T
e. T

The dose is 1–2 mg IV.

**Q.2.20  Activated charcoal:**

   a.  Is a non-specific adsorbent
   b.  Is indicated in paraquat poisoning
   c.  Is useful in tricyclic antidepressant poisoning
   d.  Is given in salicylate poisoning
   e.  May be put down the gastric tube

**Q.2.21  The following analgesics inhibit the release and dispersal of prostaglandins:**

   a.  Aspirin
   b.  Codeine
   c.  Paracetamol
   d.  Ibuprofen
   e.  Morphine

**For answers see over**

# Answers

**A.2.20**  a.  T
          b.  T
          c.  T
          d.  F
          e.  T

The dosage is Medicoal 1–2 sachets every 20 minutes or Carbomix 25–50 g every 4 hours. Carbomix may cause severe constipation and may become impacted. Medicoal is effervescent; it may cause diarrhoea but is preferable to Carbomix.

**A.2.21**  a.  T
          b.  F
          c.  T
          d.  T
          e.  F

# 3. Injury

**Q.3.1    Injury in the UK:**

a. Is the main cause of death under the age of 40 years
b. Is responsible for 18 000 deaths per year
c. Accounts for 2.6% of all causes of death
d. Causes 8%–10% of the population to attend Accident and Emergency Departments
e. Due to road traffic accidents peaks between 17.00 and 19.00 hours and 23.00 and 02.00 hours

**Q.3.2    Chest injury management involves:**

a. The airway and ventilation
b. Relieving tension pneumothorax
c. Arresting haemorrhage
d. Removal of protruding foreign bodies
e. Packing a sucking wound

**Q.3.3    A flail segment in chest injury:**

a. May be unilateral
b. May be bilateral
c. Moves outwards on inspiration
d. May compromise ventilation
e. Can be fixed with a metal plate behind the sternum

**Q.3.4    A fractured sternum:**

a. Is produced by considerable force or deceleration injury
b. Is oblique or longitudinal
c. Is an indication for ECG
d. Is extremely painful
e. Is treated by internal fixation with a Steinmann pin

**Q.3.5    A fractured rib:**

a. May cause a pneumothorax
b. May cause a haemopneumothorax
c. Is associated with blood loss
d. Is treated by binding the chest wall
e. May be treated by nerve block if pain is severe, or by local infiltration of the fracture site with lignocaine

**For answers see over**

# Answers

**A.3.1**  a. T
         b. T
         c. T
         d. T
         e. T

**A.3.2**  a. T
         b. T
         c. T
         d. F
         e. T

Protruding foreign bodies of the chest should be removed only in the operating theatre.

**A.3.3**  a. T
         b. T
         c. F
         d. T
         e. T

A flail segment results from multiple rib fractures. It is unilateral with double fractures of several ribs, bilateral with fractures of three or more ribs on both sides. The flail segment moves inwards on inspiration; this is paradoxical movement which compromises ventilation by reducing tidal volume.

**A.3.4**  a. T
         b. F
         c. T
         d. T
         e. T

The fractures are transverse, and the overlap may cause excruciating pain. Cardiac contusion may occur.

**A.3.5**  a. T
         b. T
         c. T
         d. F
         e. T

A single rib fracture may be associated with a blood loss of up to 150 ml.

**Q.3.6** **Cardiac tamponade:**

a. Is commonly due to a penetrating injury such as a knife wound
b. May result from ruptured myocardial infarction
c. Is characterised by high venous pressure
d. Is characterised by an arterial pulse which diminishes or disappears on expiration
e. Is confirmed by an increased cardiac outline on chest X-ray

**Q.3.7** **Abdominal viscera injury:**

a. Is certain if there is an imprint of clothing or tyre on the skin of the abdomen
b. May result in alteration of the abdominal contour
c. Is certain if bowel sounds are absent
d. Should be suspected if there is tenderness of the left hypochondrium
e. Should be suspected if ribs 9, 10 and 11 on the left side are fractured

**Q.3.8** **In abdominal injury peritoneal lavage:**

a. Has an accuracy of 80%–90% in diagnosing intra-abdominal bleeding
b. Should be preceded by urethral catheterisation
c. Should be performed by inserting the cannula 3–4 cm below the umbilicus
d. Need not be a cut-down procedure
e. Is performed by running in 1 litre of warm 0.9% saline with the patient in the head-down position for 10 minutes prior to peritoneal lavage drainage

**For answers see over**

# Answers

**A.3.6**  a. T
      b. T
      c. T
      d. F
      e. F

The neck veins are engorged.

The volume of the arterial pulse diminishes or disappears on inspiration. An intra-arterial line is inserted and the respiratory fluctuations observed on the oscilloscope. The cardiac silhouette may be normal on X-ray. As little as 200 ml blood in the pericardium may produce tamponade.

**A.3.7**  a. T
      b. T
      c. F
      d. T
      e. T

An imprint on the abdomen from clothing or a tyre is a reliable sign of abdominal viscera injury.

Bowel sounds may be absent in the injured patient without abdominal involvement.

Local tenderness of the left hypochondrium is suggestive of splenic rupture.

Ribs 9, 10 and 11 overlie the spleen and if fractured may be associated with rupture of the spleen.

**A.3.8**  a. T
      b. T
      c. T
      d. F
      e. T

**Q.3.9** **In stab wounds of the abdomen:**

    a. Laparotomy is mandatory if the full thickness of the abdominal wall is involved

    b. Shock and peritonitis always ensue

    c. A conservative approach may be adopted

    d. The negative laparotomy rate is well over 50%

    e. The incidence of visceral injury is 30%–40%

**Q.3.10** **Military anti-shock trousers (MAST):**

    a. Are effective in some types of shock

    b. Act by tamponade

    c. Act by autotransfusion of fluid

    d. Are useful for splinting a fractured pelvis

    e. Should be inflated to 100–110 mmHg

**Q.3.11** **Wound infection may be prevented:**

    a. By adequate surgical toilet of the wound

    b. By excision of damaged tissue

    c. By wound closure if appropriate

    d. By antibiotic therapy

    e. By routinely administering tetanus toxoid

**Q.3.12** **Gas gangrene:**

    a. Is due to contamination of a wound with *Clostridia* spores

    b. Is associated with reduced oxygen tension in the tissues

    c. Causes toxaemia by an exotoxin, lecithinase

    d. Is treated by excision of necrotic tissue

    e. Is treated with penicillin and hyperbaric oxygen

**Q.3.13** **In compound fractures:**

    a. Routine antibiotics are not indicated

    b. Anaerobe infection is unlikely

    c. Gram-positive infection is common

    d. Gas gangrene may ensue

    e. Tetanus toxoid must be given

**For answers see over**

# Answers

**A.3.9**   a. F
      b. F
      c. T
      d. F
      e. T

The patient is carefully monitored. If there is no clinical evidence of shock or peritonitis, then conservative treatment may continue.

The negative laparotomy rate has fallen from 50% to 10% with no increase in mortality.

**A.3.10**   a. T
       b. T
       c. F
       d. T
       e. F

When the trousers are correctly applied the blood supply to the lower limbs is reduced or occluded; thus there is a redistribution of cardiac output.

Low inflation pressures of 30–60 mmHg are adequate.

MAST are useful as a temporary measure and during patient transfer. They are not recommended as a substitute for transfusion.

**A.3.11**   a. T
       b. T
       c. T
       d. T
       e. T

**A.3.12**   a. T
       b. T
       c. T
       d. T
       e. T

**A.3.13**   a. F
       b. F
       c. T
       d. T
       e. T

**Q.3.14  Whiplash injury of the neck:**

  a.  Is common in rear-end traffic collisions
  b.  Is worse if there is a rotational element
  c.  May precipitate an acute disc lesion
  d.  May precipitate a dislocated mandible
  e.  Is treated by immobilisation in a soft cervical collar followed by physiotherapy

**Q.3.15  Fractured clavicle:**

  a.  Results from a fall on the flexed arm
  b.  Occurs at the junction of the proximal third and middle of the clavicle
  c.  Usually requires reduction
  d.  Is best treated with a figure-of-eight bandage
  e.  May result in mal-union

**Q.3.16  Brachial plexus lesions may:**

  a.  Result from traction injury
  b.  Result from dislocation of the shoulder or an energetic reduction
  c.  Involve the serratus anterior muscle
  d.  Produce a constricted pupil on the same side
  e.  Result from birth injury

**Q.3.17  Erb–Duchenne brachial plexus injury is characterised by:**

  a.  A lesion of the upper trunk (C5 and C6)
  b.  Paralysis of the deltoid
  c.  Paralysis of the biceps
  d.  Anaesthesia of the inner arm
  e.  Involvement of the rotators of the shoulder joint

**Q.3.18  Klumpke lower arm brachial plexus injury is characterised by:**

  a.  Lower trunk involvement (C8 –T1)
  b.  Paralysis of the extensors of the wrist
  c.  Horner's syndrome
  d.  Paralysis of the intrinsic muscles of the hand
  e.  Anaesthesia of the forearm and hand

**For answers see over**

# Answers

**A.3.14**  a.  T
         b.  T
         c.  T
         d.  T
         e.  T

**A.3.15**  a.  F
         b.  F
         c.  F
         d.  F
         e.  T

Fractured clavicle results from a fall on the outstretched arm and the site is usually the junction of the middle and distal third of the clavicle. It is best treated by the application of a broad arm sling.

**A.3.16**  a.  T
         b.  T
         c.  F
         d.  T
         e.  T

**A.3.17**  a.  T
         b.  T
         c.  T
         d.  F
         e.  T

The arm is internally rotated by the unopposed subscapularis muscle and hangs by the side with the forearm pronated in the "tip" position.

**A.3.18**  a.  T
         b.  F
         c.  T
         d.  T
         e.  T

The lower nerve trunk may be injured by inclusion with the subclavian artery in a ligature, or with an unreduced dislocation of the head of the humerus.

There may be a history of the patient clutching at an object whilst falling, and hyperabducting the arm.

**Q.3.19** **Radial nerve injury:**

a. Usually results from fracture of the upper shaft of the humerus
b. Causes paralysis of the biceps muscle
c. Causes paralysis of the extensor muscles of the wrist and fingers with wrist drop
d. Produces anaesthesia of the forearm
e. Causes inability to extend the terminal phalanges

**Q.3.20** **Median nerve injury:**

a. Occurs usually at the wrist with severed flexor tendons
b. Results in paralysis of opponens pollicis and abductor pollicis muscles
c. Results in wasting of the thenar eminence
d. Results in paralysis of all the lumbrical muscles
e. Causes loss of sensation of the thumb, index and middle fingers and the lateral palm of the hand

**Q.3.21** **Ulnar nerve injury:**

a. Usually occurs at the elbow and is associated with fracture or dislocation
b. May result also from a wrist wound
c. Results in main en griffe deformity
d. Results in wasting between the metacarpals and the hypothenar eminence
e. Rarely produces loss of sensation

**For answers see over**

# Answers

**A.3.19**  a.  T
           b.  F
           c.  T
           d.  F
           e.  F

The triceps muscle is paralysed.

There is practically no loss of sensation.

The terminal phalanges can still be extended by the interossei and lumbrical muscles.

Crutch palsy from injury in the axilla is less common now that crutches have hand grips.

**A.3.20**  a.  T
           b.  T
           c.  T
           d.  F
           e.  T

Opposition of the thumb towards the little finger may be simulated by the use of the unparalysed flexor and adductor pollicis muscles.

The outer two lumbrical muscles are affected.

The loss of sensation of the dorsum of the hand is limited to the terminal two-thirds of the middle and index finger and terminal half of the thumb.

When the median nerve is injured at the elbow the pronators and the majority of the flexors of the wrist and fingers are all paralysed.

**A.3.21**  a.  T
           b.  T
           c.  T
           d.  T
           e.  F

There is paralysis of the interossei and inner two lumbrical muscles, adductor pollicis and hypothenar muscles. Loss of sensation occurs over the medial part of the hand, palm and dorsum and includes the little finger and medial part of the ring finger.

**Q.3.22   Volkmann's ischaemic contracture:**

a. Is a complication of supracondylar fracture
b. Is due to a haematoma compressing the brachial artery
c. Results in shortening of the flexor muscles due to fibrosis
d. Results in flexion of the wrist
e. May be confirmed by flexing the wrist, and the fingers can often be extended

**Q.3.23   Fracture of the fifth metacarpal:**

a. Results from direct violence
b. Is often self-inflicted
c. May result in rotation of the little finger
d. Can be treated by neighbour-strapping with Micropore of the ring and little fingers
e. May be unstable; internal fixation with a Kirschner wire is then indicated

**Q.3.24   Torn cartilage of the knee:**

a. Is a common football injury
b. Causes the knee to be locked in extension
c. Is commoner in the lateral meniscus than the medial
d. Is accompanied by an effusion
e. Is tender over the meniscus

**Q.3.25   Rupture of the Achilles tendon:**

a. Usually occurs at the insertion
b. Causes inability to dorsiflex the foot
c. Is painful and is preceded by a feeling of being struck in the calf from behind
d. Is best examined with the patient lying prone or kneeling on a chair
e. May be treated by tendon repair or immobilisation in plaster of Paris

**For answers see over**

# Answers

**A.3.22**  a.  T
          b.  T
          c.  T
          d.  T
          e.  T

**A.3.23**  a.  T
          b.  T
          c.  T
          d.  T
          e.  T

Such fractures are often caused by karate, or punching a wall.

Rotation of the little finger often ensues.

**A.3.24**  a.  T
          b.  F
          c.  F
          d.  T
          e.  T

The knee is locked in flexion.

The lateral meniscus is torn less commonly than the medial as it is more mobile and less adherent to the capsule.

**A.3.25**  a.  F
          b.  F
          c.  T
          d.  T
          e.  T

The site is usually over 5 cm proximal to the insertion.

It causes inability to plantarflex the foot. The patient is unable to stand on tip-toes. The patient is examined prone with the feet extending over the edge of the couch or kneeling with the feet extending over the edge of the chair. The gap may be palpable if there is no swelling. Squeezing the calf causes no plantar flexion response.

**Q.3.26** **Regarding ankle sprains:**

a. Deltoid ligament sprains are commoner than lateral ligament sprains
b. Inability to bear weight on the affected limb is an indication for X-ray
c. Swelling alone is a reliable indicator of injury severity
d. The treatment is physiotherapy
e. The treatment is the application of wool and a crêpe bandage

**Q.3.27** **Metatarsal fractures:**

a. Result from falling forwards
b. Result from a heavy weight falling on the foot
c. Require no treatment
d. Should be treated with a wool and crêpe bandage
e. Should be treated by the application of a below-knee walking plaster of Paris cast

**Q.3.28** **Can shock be:**

a. Hypovolaemic
b. Cardiogenic
c. Septic
d. Anaphylactic
e. Neurogenic

**For answers see over**

# Answers

**A.3.26**  a. F
          b. T
          c. F
          d. T
          e. F

Inversion injuries or lateral ligament sprains are far commoner than eversion or deltoid ligament sprains. Three to five per cent of patients attending Accident and Emergency Departments have inversion sprains; most of these are young people.

Physiotherapy consists of the application of ice packs followed by megapulse. A tubular support bandage is applied. A wool and crêpe bandage tends to slip, causes wrinkling of the skin and is difficult for the patient to reapply.

**A.3.27**  a. F
          b. T
          c. F
          d. F
          e. T

**A.3.28**  a. T
          b. T
          c. T
          d. T
          e. T

Shock is a complex pathophysiological process initiated by altered haemodynamic function and producing poor tissue perfusion. Inadequate tissue oxygenation and accumulation of waste products impair normal cellular metabolism, leading to circulatory failure, organ failure and death.

**Q.3.29** **Hypovolaemic shock is due to:**

    a. Blood loss – external or concealed
    b. Plasma loss in burns
    c. Excessive vomiting
    d. Acute diarrhoea
    e. Multiple trauma

**Q.3.30** **Adult respiratory distress syndrome (ARDS):**

    a. Is the pulmonary component of multi-system organ failure
    b. Has a mortality of 50%
    c. Has a mortality of around 90% if there is septicaemia
    d. May be caused by trauma
    e. May be aggravated by antibiotics

**For answers see over**

# *Answers*

**A.3.29**  a. T
        b. T
        c. T
        d. T
        e. T

Unless the haemorrhage is massive the initial haematocrit is usually normal.

A female patient presenting with hypovolaemic shock with no history of injury should be regarded as having a ruptured ectopic pregnancy.

**A.3.30**  a. T
        b. T
        c. T
        d. T
        e. F

## The Injury Severity Score (ISS) and Abbreviated Injury Scale (AIS)

The Injury Severity Score (ISS) is determined by adding the squares of the highest Abbreviated Injury Scale (AIS) in each of the most severely injured body regions.

*AIS severity codes (1–6):*

1. Minor
2. Moderate
3. Serious
4. Severe
5. Critical
6. Virtually unsurvivable

An ISS of 75 is the highest possible. Injuries coded AIS 6 are automatically assigned an ISS of 75.

*Body regions:*

External
Head or neck
Face
Chest
Abdomen
Extremities

*Example 1*

A motorcyclist brought into the resuscitation area with a fractured base of skull, a fractured femur and a laceration of the arms would have an ISS of 19:

| | | |
|---|---|---|
| Fractured base of skull | AIS 3 | Region: Head/neck |
| Fractured femur | AIS 3 | Region: Extremities |
| Laceration of arms | AIS 1 | Region: External |

*Example 2*

A patient with a burn of surface area 30%–39% would have an ISS of 16:

| | | |
|---|---|---|
| Burns | AIS 4 | Region: External |

## Priorities in the Resuscitation Room

**A**    Airway/suction

**B**    Bag/intubation/oxygen

**C**    Cardioversion
     Central venous pressure
     Chest drain

**D**    Degrees – temperature
     Dextrose

**E**    Eyes – pupils

**F**    Firm collar
     Fracture splints

**G**    Group + cross-match
     Blood gases
     Glasgow Coma Scale

**H**    Haemorrhage

**I**    IV line – subclavian
     Infusion – crystalloid/colloid

**J**    Joules

**K**    KG – ECG

**L**    Lateral + AP cervical X-ray; skull X-ray; upright chest X-ray

**M**    Monitor
     MAST

**N**    Naloxone

**O**    Oro/nasogastric tube
     Optic fundi

**P**    Pass urethral catheter
     Peritoneal lavage

**Q**    Question ambulance crew/witnesses/relatives

**R**    Record drugs, dose, time on white board

**S**    Scan

**T**    Transfer only when stable

# 4. Burns

**Q.4.1** **In an extensively burned patient:**

    a. The plasma volume falls
    b. The total blood volume falls
    c. The haematocrit falls
    d. Shock is present
    e. The patient's life is in danger

**Q.4.2** **A patient weighing 75 kg with a 50% burn requires in the first 4 hours:**

    a. 1 litre of plasma
    b. $1\frac{1}{2}$ litres of plasma
    c. $2\frac{1}{2}$ litres of plasma
    d. $3\frac{1}{2}$ litres of plasma
    e. 4 litres of plasma

**For answers see over**

# Answers

**A.4.1**  a. T
        b. T
        c. F
        d. T
        e. T

The haematocrit level progressively rises and will be around 70% when half the plasma volume is lost. In an extensive burn this may occur within 3 or 4 hours.

**A.4.2**  a. F
        b. F
        c. T
        d. F
        e. F

---

Classify into partial thickness and full thickness burns:
Partial thickness burns are painful, are hyperaesthesic to sterile pin-prick, and the removal of hair follicles with sterile tweezers is painful. Analgesia is required.
Full thickness burns are painless, are hypoaesthesic to pin-prick and removal of hair follicles is painless. Analgesia is not required.
Measure extent of burns: Rule of 9's or Lund and Browder chart.
Intravenous infusion is indicated if 15% burns sustained in adults and 10% in children.
Calculate the fluid required over the first 4 hours after the burn:

$$\frac{\text{Amount required}}{\text{per unit time (ml)}} = \frac{\text{Percentage area of burn} \times \text{weight in kg}}{2}$$

Equal volumes of fluid are transfused in unit time in hours

| 4 | 4 | 4 | 6 | 6 | 12 |

---

**Q.4.3** **Fluid therapy should consist of:**

a. Sodium solution
b. Dextrose
c. Crystalloid
d. Colloid
e. Plasma

**Q.4.4** **Ringer's solution contains:**

a. Sodium
b. Chloride
c. Potassium
d. Bicarbonate
e. Calcium

**Q.4.5** **With regard to colloid infusion:**

a. One-third of the volume is required compared with crystalloid infusion
b. The risk of tissue oedema is low
c. Polygeline has a lower sodium content than Gelofusine
d. Gelofusine has a higher calcium content than Polygeline
e. Shelf-life of colloids is short

**Q.4.6** **The total body sodium content is:**

a. 1000 mmol
b. 3000 mmol
c. 5000 mmol
d. 7000 mmol
e. 10 000 mmol

**For answers see over**

# Answers

**A.4.3**   a.  T
           b.  F
           c.  T
           d.  T
           e.  T

A sodium-free solution can cause death by intracellular overhydration (water intoxication).

Five per cent dextrose is metabolised and becomes solute free. Water thus enters the cells producing intracellular oedema.

Ringer's solution is a satisfactory crystalloid but only one-quarter remains in the circulation; the rest fills the extravascular interstitial space.

Infusion may begin with Ringer's solution followed by a colloid: Polygeline, Gelofusine or Hetastarch.

Human plasma protein fraction solution (HPPF) is the most appropriate infusion and better than freeze-dried plasma. Plasma remains in the circulation. Hetastarch 6% (Hespan) is a good alternative to HPPF and cheaper. The colloidal properties approximate those of human albumin.

**A.4.4**   a.  T
           b.  T
           c.  T
           d.  F
           e.  T

**A.4.5**   a.  T
           b.  T
           c.  T
           d.  F
           e.  F

**A.4.6**   a.  F
           b.  F
           c.  T
           d.  F
           e.  F

**Q.4.7** The plasma bicarbonate level is:

    a. 11–15 mEq/l
    b. 16–21 mEq/l
    c. 22–25 mEq/l
    d. 26–31 mEq/l
    e. 32–35 mEq/l

**Q.4.8** The management of superficial burns over 20% of the body surface includes:

    a. Analgesia
    b. Infusion of crystalloid
    c. Haematocrit readings
    d. Tetanus toxoid
    e. Exposure

**Q.4.9** The management of extensive deep burns over 50% of the body surface includes:

    a. Morphine
    b. Infusion of crystalloid
    c. Infusion of colloid
    d. Infusion of plasma
    e. Monitoring urinary output

**Q.4.10** Analgesia is always indicated in:

    a. Flash burns
    b. Scalds
    c. Petrol burns
    d. Paraffin burns
    e. Hydrofluoric acid burns

**Q.4.11** In the management of bitumen burns:

    a. Analgesia is usually required
    b. The bitumen should be removed
    c. Cold water is useful
    d. The blisters should be left
    e. The burns should be dressed

**For answers see over**

**A.4.7**  a. F
        b. F
        c. T
        d. F
        e. F

**A.4.8**  a. T
        b. T
        c. T
        d. T
        e. T

**A.4.9**  a. F
        b. T
        c. T
        d. T
        e. T

**A.4.10**  a. T
        b. T
        c. F
        d. F
        e. T

When analgesia is indicated Entonox is of value.

When morphine is required give 0.1 mg/kg body weight IV.

Tetanus toxoid should be given routinely.

**A.4.11**  a. T
        b. F
        c. T
        d. F
        e. T

Cold water should be applied liberally.

Bitumen remover should not be used; the bitumen should be left and the burns dressed. The bitumen can be removed with the blisters.

**Q.4.12  Hydrofluoric acid burns:**

  a.  Are usually small
  b.  Are extremely painful
  c.  May cause hypocalcaemia
  d.  Can be treated with Flamazine
  e.  Should be exposed

**Q.4.13  Electrical burns:**

  a.  Usually affect the fingers
  b.  May appear small and innocuous
  c.  Exhibit small areas of necrotic skin
  d.  Always involve underlying tissue
  e.  Frequently involve tendons

**Q.4.14  Smoke inhalation:**

  a.  Is characterised by tachycardia
  b.  Is characterised by tachypnoea
  c.  Is characterised by a fall in $pO_2$
  d.  Should be treated with a nebuliser of salbutamol
  e.  Should be treated with 100% oxygen

**For answers see over**

**A.4.12**  a. T
          b. T
          c. T
          d. F
          e. F

The fingers are usually affected.

The burns are extremely painful and analgesia is required.

Absorption causes hypocalcaemia.

Treatment is 2.5% calcium gluconate gel applied liberally four times per day. Ten per cent solution may be injected beneath the burn area.

**A.4.13**  a. T
          b. T
          c. T
          d. T
          e. T

**A.4.14**  a. T
          b. T
          c. T
          d. T
          e. T

Chest X-ray may reveal pneumothorax or pulmonary oedema.

The fumes may be toxic due to cyanates and may be hot. Burns around the mouth indicate burns of the upper and possibly lower respiratory tract.

# 5.  *Some Joints and Some Orthopaedics*

**Q.5.1** **An acute hot swollen knee may be due to:**

a. Tuberculosis
b. Gonorrhoea
c. Typhoid fever
d. Pneumococcal septicaemia
e. Diphtheria

**Q.5.2** **Rheumatoid arthritis:**

a. Affects men more than women
b. Starts in the synovial membrane
c. Affects the terminal phalanges of the fingers
d. May cause flexion and ulnar deviation of the wrist
e. May be associated with anaemia

**Q.5.3** **In ankylosing spondylitis:**

a. More women suffer from the disease than men
b. The age group is 15–40 years
c. The erythrocyte sedimentation rate is raised
d. Iridocyclitis is common
e. Aortic incompetence may occur

**Q.5.4** **Sjögren's syndrome is characterised by:**

a. Epiphora
b. Psoriasis
c. Rheumatoid arthritis
d. Dry mouth
e. A wide range of auto-antibodies

**Q.5.5** **The neuropathic joint:**

a. Affects the knee in tabes dorsalis
b. Affects the shoulder in syringomyelia
c. May be seen in the foot in diabetes mellitus
d. Is painful
e. Is characterised by gross deformity and hypermobility

**For answers see over**

# Answers

**A.5.1**  a. F
b. T
c. T
d. T
e. F

**A.5.2**  a. F
b. T
c. F
d. T
e. T

**A.5.3**  a. F
b. T
c. T
d. T
e. T

**A.5.4**  a. F
b. F
c. T
d. T
e. T

Sjögren's syndrome is a connective tissue disorder with xerostomia and keratoconjunctivitis sicca.

**A.5.5**  a. T
b. T
c. T
d. F
e. T

**Q.5.6    Gout:**

    a. Is a disorder of purine metabolism
    b. Commonly affects the big toe
    c. In the hand is called cheiragra
    d. May present as tophi in the ears
    e. Cannot be diagnosed by X-ray

**Q.5.7    The painful arc syndrome of the shoulder:**

    a. Is characterised by pain on abduction 60°–120°
    b. Is painless above or below this arc
    c. May be due to subacromial bursitis
    d. May be due to inflammation or degeneration of the supra spinatus tendon
    e. Is periarthritis

**Q.5.8    Frozen shoulder:**

    a. Is common in young people
    b. Is worse during the day time
    c. May result from immobilisation
    d. May restrict movement to scapulo-thoracic
    e. Is capsulitis

**Q.5.9    Thoracic inlet syndrome:**

    a. May be due to a cervical rib
    b. May be due to pressure by the scalenus anterior muscle
    c. May be due to stretching of the plexus over the first rib
    d. Is characterised by pain and paraesthesia
    e. Is commonly seen in men

**For answers see over**

# Answers

**A.5.6**    a.  T
          b.  T
          c.  T
          d.  T
          e.  F

The gouty tophi (from the Latin *gutta*, a drop, and *tophus*, a rock) are deposits of sodium biurate.

Clear translucent areas due to the presence of sodium biurate may be seen in the heads of the phalanges on X-ray.

Distinguishing gout from other acute monoarthroses and joint sepsis may be difficult. The blood uric acid may not be helpful (normal level 0.1–0.4 mmol/l). Only the isolation of urate crystals in the aspirate is conclusive diagnosis.

**A.5.7**    a.  T
          b.  T
          c.  T
          d.  T
          e.  F

**A.5.8**    a.  F
          b.  F
          c.  T
          d.  T
          e.  T

The age group is 50–60.

Pain in the deltoid region interferes with sleep.

**A.5.9**    a.  T
          b.  T
          c.  T
          d.  T
          e.  F

**Q.5.10    Thoracic inlet syndrome:**

a. May affect the small muscles of the hand
b. May affect the subclavian artery
c. May produce coldness and pallor of the hand
d. Is worse at night
e. Can be confused with the carpal tunnel syndrome

**Q.5.11    The carpal tunnel syndrome:**

a. Is due to compression of the ulnar nerve
b. Occurs in early pregnancy
c. Occurs in rheumatoid arthritis
d. Is characterised by night pain
e. May produce wasting of the thumb muscles

**Q.5.12    Tennis elbow is:**

a. Medial epicondylitis
b. Olecranon bursitis
c. Supinator myositis ossificans
d. Pain in the lateral epicondyle
e. Pain at the attachment of flexor muscles

**Q.5.13    Pulled elbow:**

a. Occurs in a child suspended by the arm, usually by an impatient person
b. Is characterised by pain and stiffness
c. Is characterised by inability to pronate
d. Produces a fat pad sign on X ray
e. Is treated by supinating the forearm

**For answers see over**

**A.5.10**  a. T
         b. T
         c. T
         d. T
         e. T

Women are more often affected than men. Some women complain of weakness and coldness of the hand on fastening their bra behind the back. This results from subclavian artery compression.

**A.5.11**  a. F
         b. T
         c. T
         d. T
         e. T

The pain occurs in the distribution of the median nerve and is due to compression by the transverse carpal ligament of the wrist.

**A.5.12**  a. F
         b. F
         c. F
         d. T
         e. F

**A.5.13**  a. T
         b. T
         c. F
         d. F
         e. T

The child is unable to supinate the forearm.

The X-ray is normal.

**Q.5.14  March fracture:**

a. Is common
b. Involves the second or third metatarsal
c. Is preceded by injury
d. Is often associated with excessive walking
e. Is always confirmed by X-ray

**Q.5.15  Acute pain down the arm may be due to:**

a. Acute traction injury
b. Acute myocardial infarction
c. Acute cervical disc
d. Cervical spondylosis
e. Acute radiculitis

**Q.5.16  In prolapsed intervertebral lumbar disc:**

a. There is acute sciatic pain
b. There may be radiation to the foot
c. The ankle jerk is increased
d. There is pain on lowering the elevated limb
e. There may be tenderness of L5–S1

**For answers see over**

# Answers

**A.5.14**  a. T
           b. T
           c. F
           d. T
           e. F

Initial X-ray may reveal a hair-line fracture or may be normal. Callus may be seen 2 weeks later.

**A.5.15**  a. T
           b. T
           c. T
           d. T
           e. T

**A.5.16**  a. T
           b. T
           c. F
           d. F
           e. T

The ankle jerk is diminished or absent.

The Lasègue sign or sciatic nerve stretch test is positive on elevating the leg. Pain caused by lowering the leg should arise suspicion of psoas abscess due to tuberculous osteitis.

# 6. *Hand and Finger Lesions*

**Q.6.1** **Orf:**

a. Affects shepherds, butchers and veterinary surgeons
b. Has an incubation period of 2 weeks
c. Is non-irritant
d. Is characterised by a red-blue papule which becomes a haemorrhagic bullous
e. Should be excised


**Q.6.2** **Dermoid cyst:**

a. Is an implantation dermoid
b. Is usually due to skin trauma
c. Is yellow in colour
d. Contains sebum
e. Transilluminates


**Q.6.3** **Erysipeloid of the finger:**

a. Is an infection of the epidermis
b. Affects butchers and fishmongers
c. Is characterised by pain and swelling
d. Looks well defined and lilac-coloured
e. Is purulent


**Q.6.4** **Herpes of the finger:**

a. Curiously affects nurses
b. Presents with vesicles and cellulitis
c. Fails to respond to antibiotics
d. May resolve spontaneously
e. May be treated with idoxuridine


**For answers see over**

# Answers

**A.6.1**  a.  T
          b.  F
          c.  F
          d.  T
          e.  F

Orf is due to a virus from the mouth of sheep.

The incubation period is 5 days.

Itching is intense.

The haemorrhagic bullous ruptures becoming an umbilicated ulcer.

Spontaneous healing occurs in 3–6 weeks.

**A.6.2**  a.  T
          b.  T
          c.  T
          d.  T
          e.  F

**A.6.3**  a.  T
          b.  T
          c.  T
          d.  T
          e.  F

**A.6.4**  a.  T
          b.  T
          c.  T
          d.  T
          e.  T

### Q.6.5 A ganglion:

a. Is a myxomatous degeneration of fibrous tissue
b. Is related to tendon sheath and joint capsules
c. Is painless
d. Does not transilluminate
e. May be ruptured by external pressure

### Q.6.6 Beryllium granuloma:

a. Is seen following cuts from broken fluorescent light tubes
b. Is a wound that does not heal
c. Occurs in the hand, usually fingers
d. Is characterised by swelling and induration with central ulceration
e. Is treated by cryotherapy or surgical excision

### Q.6.7 Zirconium granuloma:

a. Occurs on hands
b. May occur in axillae from deodorants
c. Is characterised by persistent soft red-brown papules
d. Reveals tubercles without caseation
e. Has a histopathology similar to that of sarcoid

### Q.6.8 Acrylic finger-tip dermatitis:

a. Occurs in dentists and dental technicians from contact with dentures
b. Occurs in manufacturers of contact lenses
c. Occurs in manufacturers of orthopaedic prostheses
d. Is characterised by redness, oedema and vesiculation
e. Usually affects only one finger

**For answers see over**

**A.6.5**   a. T
         b. T
         c. F
         d. F
         e. T

A ganglion may become tense and painful.

It transilluminates brilliantly.

It is common in the wrist.

Hitting it with the family Bible is not recommended.

**A.6.6**   a. T
         b. T
         c. T
         d. T
         e. T

**A.6.7**   a. T
         b. T
         c. T
         d. T
         e. T

**A.6.8**   a. T
         b. T
         c. T
         d. T
         e. F

**Q.6.9** **Pulp space infection:**

    a. Causes cellulitis of fatty and areolar tissue
    b. May cause osteitis of the terminal phalanx
    c. May compress the terminal branches of digital arteries
    d. Does not include the flexor tendon
    e. Is treated by an incision over the site of maximum tenderness

**Q.6.10** **Web space infection:**

    a. Is potentially dangerous
    b. Spreads into the palmar spaces
    c. Is characterised by pain, swelling and cellulitis
    d. Is treated by incision under local anaesthesia
    e. Is treated also with flucloxacillin or penicillin

**Q.6.11** **Trigger thumb:**

    a. Is characterised by clicking
    b. Is worse at night
    c. Progresses to flexion
    d. Can be extended with difficulty
    e. May occur in infants

**Q.6.12** **de Quervain's disease is:**

    a. Pain in the thumb
    b. Tenosynovitis
    c. Localised to the radial styloid with tenderness
    d. Worse when the thumb is passively abducted
    e. A swelling which may be palpable over the tendon

**Q.6.13** **Boutonnière deformity:**

    a. Is a rupture of the central slip of the extensor expansion of the finger
    b. Adopts the therapeutic posture of the mallet finger
    c. Is characterised by flexion of the proximal interphalangeal joint
    d. Is characterised by flexion of the distal interphalangeal joint
    e. Is repaired by suturing together the two lateral slips

**For answers see over**

# *Answers*

**A.6.9** a. T
   b. T
   c. T
   d. F
   e. T

The infection may spread to the synovial sheath of the flexor tendon inserted into the base of the terminal phalanx.

**A.6.10** a. T
    b. T
    c. T
    d. F
    e. T

**A.6.11** a. T
    b. F
    c. T
    d. T
    e. T

Trigger thumb is usually worse in the morning.

**A.6.12** a. T
    b. T
    c. T
    d. F
    e. T

This is a stenosing tenosynovitis affecting the abductor pollicis longus and the extensor pollicis brevis tendons. Passive flexion across the palm accentuates the pain.

**A.6.13** a. T
    b. T
    c. T
    d. F
    e. T

### Q.6.14 Dupuytren's contracture:

a. Commonly affects the index finger
b. Commonly affects the ring finger
c. Is frequent in black races
d. May be associated with cirrhosis of the liver
e. Is relieved by excision of the palmar fascia

### Q.6.15 Degloving:

a. Commonly results from wrenching of a ring
b. Is often an industrial accident
c. May be total
d. Is routinely treated by skin graft
e. If total requires amputation of the finger

### Q.6.16 Bursting injury of the finger:

a. Is a contusion injury with laceration and tissue damage
b. Is characterised by swelling and gaping
c. Is often associated with a fractured terminal phalanx
d. Should be sutured
e. Should be dressed and examined frequently for sepsis

**For answers see over**

# Answers

**A.6.14**  a. F
        b. T
        c. F
        d. T
        e. T

**A.6.15**  a. T
        b. T
        c. T
        d. F
        e. T

**A.6.16**  a. T
        b. T
        c. T
        d. F
        e. T

Viable and non-viable tissue may be present. Exudate should be allowed to drain. Suturing is not advisable.

# 7. Fits, Faints and Weakness

**Q.7.1 Fits and faints may be due to:**

a. Epilepsy
b. Hypoglycaemia
c. Cerebral ischaemia
d. Syncope
e. Hysteria

**Q.7.2 Grand mal is characterised by:**

a. An aura
b. Unconsciousness
c. A tonic and clonic phase
d. Incontinence of urine
e. Post-epileptiform headache

**For answers see over**

# Answers

**A.7.1**   a. T
        b. T
        c. T
        d. T
        e. T

All patients with epilepsy should have a blood sugar examination.

Hypoglycaemia is often due to insulin overdosage as the result of mismeasurement in the insulin-dependent diabetic. It also occurs in the elderly diabetic on oral therapy. Hypoglycaemia may also be due to an insulinoma of the pancreas. Such patients are often misdiagnosed for years and treated as having epilepsy. The majority of insulinomas are benign and operable.

Transient cerebral ischaemic attacks may be due to vertebrobasilar artery insufficiency as a result of stenosis of the vertebral or subclavian artery.

Adams–Stokes attacks are due to complete heart block and occur when the heart rate is below 30 per minute. The attack may be followed by an anoxic convulsion. A cannon 'a' wave is seen in the jugular venous pulse. On auscultation there is changing intensity and alteration of the first heart sound.

Syncope from a simple faint may result from an unpleasant experience, sight or smell. Syncope may occur at the onset of an attack of supraventricular tachycardia. Micturition syncope occurs in elderly men getting out of bed at night. This may be confused with nocturnal epilepsy.

**A.7.2**   a. T
        b. T
        c. T
        d. T
        e. T

In patients on long-term phenytoin therapy hyperplasia of the gums develops – a useful physical sign if no history is available and the fit was unwitnessed. There may also be scars of the tongue.

The EEG consists of multiple high-voltage spikes, widespread and synchronous in both hemispheres.

**Q.7.3** **Petit mal is characterised by:**

a. Brief loss of consciousness
b. Convulsion
c. Incontinence
d. Confusion after the attack
e. Characteristic EEG

**Q.7.4** **The patient with temporal lobe epilepsy:**

a. May present with gustatory aura
b. May present with perceptional illusions
c. Has *déjà vu*
d. Has uncinate attacks
e. Has a typical EEG

**Q.7.5** **Subclavian steal syndrome is characterised by:**

a. Vertigo
b. Drop attacks
c. A loud bruit in the neck
d. Normal radial pulse
e. Normal angiography

For answers see over

# Answers

**A.7.3**    a.  T
            b.  F
            c.  F
            d.  F
            e.  T

The unconsciousness may last only a few seconds.

The patient does not fall or convulse.

After the attack he/she continues as though nothing had happened.

The EEG records 3 per second wave and spike synchronous over both frontal lobes.

**A.7.4**    a.  T
            b.  T
            c.  T
            d.  T
            e.  T

The gustatory aura may be followed by automatic movements of chewing and smacking of the lips – uncinate attacks. The patient looks dazed and does not respond when addressed. There may be disordered awareness.

*Déjà vu* is common.

The EEG reveals focal sharp and slow waves in the temporal region.

Carbamazepine is the drug of choice in controlling temporal lobe seizures.

**A.7.5**    a.  T
            b.  T
            c.  T
            d.  F
            e.  F

The radial pulse on the affected side may be absent.

Symptoms are due to reversal of blood down the vertebral artery on the affected side causing brain ischaemia.

Arch angiography reveals stenosis or occlusion of the subclavian or innominate artery proximal to the origin of the vertebral artery.

**Q.7.6    Other causes of fits and faints include:**

a. Narcolepsy
b. Tetany
c. Apnoea
d. Trauma
e. Postural hypotension

**Q.7.7    Narcolepsy:**

a. Is common
b. Is characterised by constant sleepiness
c. Is often diagnosed as hysteria
d. May be diagnosed as neurasthenia
e. Is treated with amphetamine

**Q.7.8    Tetany:**

a. Is an increased excitability of peripheral nerves
b. Is due to low plasma calcium
c. Is due to alkalosis
d. Produces carpopedal spasm
e. Produces stridor

**For answers see over**

# Answers

**A.7.6**  a. T
         b. T
         c. T
         d. T
         e. T

Post-traumatic epilepsy occurs in 5% of head injuries admitted to hospital.

**A.7.7**  a. F
         b. F
         c. T
         d. T
         e. T

The condition is rare but not infrequently diagnosed.

The patient has an irresistible attack of sleep, often in inappropriate circumstances, from which he/she can be aroused immediately.

**A.7.8**  a. T
         b. T
         c. T
         d. T
         e. T

Depletion of plasma calcium is caused by hypoparathyroidism, rickets, osteomalacia, malabsorption syndrome and chronic renal failure.

Alakalosis is caused by repeated vomiting, excessive absorbable alkalis, hyperventilation and primary aldosteronism.

In children a triad occurs: stridor, carpopedal spasm (main d'accoucheur) and convulsions. Adults may complain of tingling around the mouth, and hands and feet, or painful carpopedal spasm.

Latent tetany may be detected by Trousseau's sign.

Tetany due to low plasma calcium is treated with 20 ml 10% calcium gluconate IV. Alkalotic tetany due to persistent vomiting is best treated with an infusion of isotonic saline. Hyperventilation tetany is treated by making the patient rebreathe into a paper bag.

**Q.7.9    Blood pressure which falls on standing up:**

a. Is orthostatic hypotension
b. May be due to drugs
c. Is significant if the fall is 10–15 mmHg
d. Usually occurs in the morning
e. Affects the middle-aged and elderly

**Q.7.10   Weakness may be due to:**

a. Carcinomatosis
b. Post-viral fatigue syndrome
c. Addison's disease
d. Primary aldosteronism
e. Myasthenia gravis

**Q.7.11   Post-viral fatigue syndrome:**

a. Is myalgic encephalitis
b. Follows influenza, sore throat or glandular fever
c. Is characterised by weakness
d. Has been called Yuppie flu
e. Is hysteria

**Q.7.12   Addison's disease:**

a. Is more common in males
b. Affects the adrenal medulla
c. Is autoimmune failure
d. May be due to tuberculosis
e. Causes adrenocortical antibodies to be present in the serum

**For answers see over**

# Answers

**A.7.9**   a. T
           b. T
           c. F
           d. T
           e. T

It is clinically significant if the fall in systolic blood pressure is 30 mmHg or more.

**A.7.10**   a. T
           b. T
           c. T
           d. T
           e. T

**A.7.11**   a. T
           b. T
           c. T
           d. T
           e. F

The post-viral fatigue syndrome came to light in 1955 in an outbreak at the Royal Free Hospital in London and was dismissed as hysterical. Some nurses were accused of malingering. It is due to lingering infection by the enterovirus group.

**A.7.12**   a. F
           b. F
           c. T
           d. T
           e. T

Females are affected twice as frequently as males.

There is atrophy of the cells of the three layers of the adrenal cortex.

**Q.7.13   Addison's disease is characterised by:**

    a. Weakness
    b. Weight loss
    c. Pigmentation
    d. Gastrointestinal disorder
    e. Low blood pressure

**Q.7.14   Aldosteronism:**

    a. Is primary or secondary
    b. Is overactivity of the zona fasciculata/reticularis
    c. Is confirmed by urinary aldosterone estimation
    d. Is confirmed by plasma aldosterone assay
    e. Is confirmed by plasma renin assay

**Q.7.15   Primary aldosteronism:**

    a. Is associated with an adenoma
    b. Is associated with episodic weakness
    c. Is associated with potassium deficiency
    d. May be associated with tetany
    e. Is associated with low blood pressure

**Q.7.16   Secondary aldosteronism:**

    a. Occurs in cirrhosis
    b. Occurs in nephrotic syndrome
    c. May be associated with renal artery stenosis
    d. Is associated with hyperkalaemia
    e. Is characterised by oedema

**Q.7.17   Myasthenia gravis:**

    a. Mainly affects facial muscles
    b. Is characterised by ptosis
    c. Is characterised by diplopia
    d. Is commoner in men than women
    e. Responds to neostigmine

**For answers see over**

# Answers

**A.7.13**  a. T
        b. T
        c. T
        d. T
        e. T

In adrenal crisis the gastrointestinal complaint may be predominant and may simulate an acute abdomen or severe gastroenteritis.

**A.7.14**  a. T
        b. F
        c. T
        d. T
        e. T

Aldosteronism is overactivity of the zona glomerulosa of the adrenal gland.

**A.7.15**  a. T
        b. T
        c. T
        d. T
        e. F

Primary aldosteronism, or Conn's syndrome, is treated by removal of the affected gland or spironolactone therapy.

**A.7.16**  a. T
        b. T
        c. T
        d. F
        e. T

**A.7.17**  a. T
        b. T
        c. T
        d. F
        e. T

# 8.  Eye Lesions

**Q.8.1** **An acute red eye signifies:**

    a. Conjunctivitis
    b. Corneal ulceration
    c. Cataract
    d. Acute glaucoma
    e. Iritis

**Q.8.2** **Vision is normal in:**

    a. Conjunctivitis
    b. Iritis
    c. Acute glaucoma
    d. Episcleritis
    e. Keratitis

**Q.8.3** **The pupil is normal in:**

    a. Conjunctivitis
    b. Iritis
    c. Acute glaucoma
    d. Episcleritis
    e. Keratitis

**Q.8.4** **The cornea is clear in:**

    a. Conjunctivitis
    b. Iritis
    c. Acute glaucoma
    d. Episcleritis
    e. Keratitis

**Q.8.5** **Photophobia is common in:**

    a. Conjunctivitis
    b. Iritis
    c. Acute glaucoma
    d. Episcleritis
    e. Keratitis

**For answers see over**

# Answers

**A.8.1**   a. T
          b. T
          c. F
          d. T
          e. T

**A.8.2**   a. T
          b. F
          c. F
          d. T
          e. T

**A.8.3**   a. T
          b. F
          c. F
          d. T
          e. T

In acute glaucoma the patient may present with vomiting. The pupil is oval and fixed, and does not react to light or consensual stimulae. The cornea is hazy, there is ciliary injection, and the eye feels hard due to increased intra-ocular tension.

**A.8.4**   a. T
          b. T
          c. F
          d. T
          e. F

**A.8.5**   a. T
          b. T
          c. F
          d. F
          e. T

**Q.8.6**  **Hyphaema is:**

    a. Haemorrhage of the anterior cranial fossa
    b. Cellulitis of the orbit
    c. Blood in the anterior chamber
    d. Blood in the frontal sinus
    e. Inflammation of subcutaneous tissues

**Q.8.7**  **Intraocular foreign bodies are:**

    a. Often metal of high velocity
    b. Caused by hammering, chiselling or grinding
    c. Seen on X-ray
    d. Removed in the Accident and Emergency Department
    e. Always referred to an ophthalmologist

**Q.8.8**  **Perforating injuries of the eye:**

    a. Are due to road traffic accidents, industrial accidents and missiles
    b. May have bleeding from the globe or hyphaema
    c. May also have facial lacerations
    d. Should be suspected if the pupil is irregular
    e. May be associated with skull fracture

**Q.8.9**  **Burns of the cornea are:**

    a. Due to acid or alkali
    b. Due to welding or sunbeds
    c. Always visible with fluorescein stain
    d. Treated with steroid drops
    e. Treated with copious irrigation, chloramphenicol drops and pad

**Q.8.10**  **Epiphora is:**

    a. Loss of smell
    b. Rhinorrhoea
    c. Unilateral loss of vision
    d. Excess of tears due to lachrymal duct obstruction
    e. Epidural infection

**For answers see over**

**A.8.6**   a.  F
          b.  F
          c.  T
          d.  F
          e.  F

**A.8.7**   a.  T
          b.  T
          c.  T
          d.  F
          e.  T

Two X-rays should be taken in the same position to exclude the possibility of an artefact on one film. A further X-ray is then taken with the patient's eyes deviated to one side.

**A.8.8**   a.  T
          b.  T
          c.  T
          d.  T
          e.  T

**A.8.9**   a.  T
          b.  T
          c.  F
          d.  F
          e.  T

Eye lavage is best done with normal saline and an infusion set. The undine is of little value.

**A.8.10**  a.  F
          b.  F
          c.  F
          d.  T
          e.  F

**Q.8.11  Proptosis may be due to:**

    a.  Cavernous sinus thrombosis
    b.  Orbital haemorrhage
    c.  Leukaemia
    d.  Orbital cellulitis
    e.  Thyrotoxicosis

**Q.8.12  Herpes simplex of the eye:**

    a.  Presents like a corneal foreign body
    b.  Is diagnosed by instillation of fluorescein
    c.  Is treated with antibiotics
    d.  Is treated with steroids
    e.  Is treated with idoxuridine

**Q.8.13  Herpes zoster of the eye:**

    a.  Is caused by the varicella zoster virus
    b.  Begins with pain in the forehead
    c.  Affects the fifth nerve
    d.  Results in a rash after 4 days
    e.  Causes swollen eyelids

**Q.8.14  Choroiditis:**

    a.  Is characterised by exudate which interrupts the vessels
    b.  May have exudate surrounded by black pigment
    c.  Is due to syphilis
    d.  Is due to sarcoidosis
    e.  Is due to toxoplasmosis

**Q.8.15  Retinitis:**

    a.  Is characterised by haemorrhages and exudates
    b.  May be associated with papilloedema
    c.  Is often due to nephritis
    d.  May be due to diabetes
    e.  May be seen in leukaemia

**For answers see over**

# Answers

**A.8.11**  a. T
           b. T
           c. T
           d. T
           e. T

**A.8.12**  a. T
           b. T
           c. F
           d. F
           e. T

**A.8.13**  a. T
           b. T
           c. T
           d. T
           e. T

**A.8.14**  a. F
           b. T
           c. T
           d. T
           e. T

**A.8.15**  a. T
           b. T
           c. T
           d. T
           e. T

The exudates interrupt the blood vessels. In albuminuric retinitis the flame-shaped haemorrhages and cotton-wool exudates are maximal at the macula.

In early diabetes dot haemorrhages or microaneurysms are seen adjacent to the capillary walls.

**Q.8.16**   **Causes of blindness in the UK include:**

    a.  Senile cataract
    b.  Macular degeneration
    c.  Retinal detachment
    d.  Glaucoma
    e.  Diabetic retinopathy

**Q.8.17**   **Causes of bilateral blindness of acute or subacute onset include:**

    a.  Injury to the occipital lobe
    b.  Methyl alcohol poisoning
    c.  Hysteria
    d.  Neuromyelitis optica
    e.  Pituitary tumour

**For answers see over**

# Answers

**A.8.16**  a.  T
           b.  T
           c.  T
           d.  T
           e.  T

**A.8.17**  a.  T
           b.  T
           c.  T
           d.  T
           e.  F

In neuromyelitis optica, transverse myelitis occurs with bilateral optic neuritis.

Pituitary tumours compress visual pathways causing visual field defects.

# 9. Child Abuse

**Q.9.1** **The following injuries in a child suggest child abuse:**

 a. Torn frenulum of the lip
 b. Small burns or bruises, particularly of the face
 c. Finger-shaped marks
 d. Subconjunctival haemorrhage
 c. Bilateral stocking burns of the ankles and feet

**Q.9.2** **Child abuse should be suspected if:**

 a. The explanation of the injury is inadequate
 b. There is evidence of previous injury
 c. There is delay between the injury and the parent seeking medical help.
 d. The child has been brought to the Accident and Emergency Department for little apparent reason
 e. A sibling has had a suspicious injury

**Q.9.3** **The abuse may be:**

 a. Physical
 b. Psychological
 c. Sexual
 d. Potential
 e. Negligent

**Q.9.4** **Sexual abuse may present as:**

 a. Injury to the genitalia
 b. Injury to the anus
 c. Recurrent urinary infection
 d. Sudden changes in behaviour
 e. Nightmares

**For answers see over**

# Answers

A.9.1    a. T
           b. T
           c. T
           d. T
           e. T

A.9.2    a. T
           b. T
           c. T
           d. T
           e. T

A.9.3    a. T
           b. T
           c. T
           d. T
           e. T

A.9.4    a. T
           b. T
           c. T
           d. T
           e. T

---

Sexual abuse affects 1 in 10 girls before the age of 16 and 1 in 15 boys before the age of 16.

Children rarely lie about sexual abuse. The majority are abused by persons related or known to them.

When child abuse is suspected the child should be admitted under the care of a paediatrician and the social services informed. A Place of Safety Order may be necessary.

# 10. *AIDS*

**Q.10.1 Acquired immune deficiency syndrome (AIDS):**

a. Is due to the human immunodeficiency virus (HIV)
b. Is due to HIV II
c. Is due to LAV II
d. Is a notifiable disease
e. Is the major cause of premature death in young men in San Francisco and New York

**Q.10.2 Transmission of HIV is by:**

a. Anal and vaginal sexual intercourse
b. Drug abusers with contaminated needles
c. Infected mother to foetus
d. Transfusion of contaminated blood
e. Skin grafts from HIV-positive donors

**Q.10.3 The virus is found in:**

a. Blood
b. Semen
c. Breast milk
d. Saliva
e. Tears

**Q.10.4 The virus is spread by:**

a. Mosquitos
b. Sharing toilets
c. Sharing cooking utensils
d. Bathing in public swimming pools
e. Coughing and sneezing

**Q.10.5 The virus is inactivated by:**

a. Cold
b. Detergents
c. Bleach
d. Glutaraldehyde 2%
e. Sodium hypochlorite 1%

**For answers see over**

# Answers

**A.10.1**  a.  T
           b.  T
           c.  T
           d.  F
           e.  T

**A.10.2**  a.  T
           b.  T
           c.  T
           d.  T
           e.  T

**A.10.3**  a.  T
           b.  T
           c.  T
           d.  T
           e.  T

Although the virus may be present in saliva, infection by this route is unlikely unless large quantities are swallowed during kissing, or if saliva is blood-stained from lip biting.

**A.10.4**  a.  F
           b.  F
           c.  F
           d.  F
           e.  F

**A.10.5**  a.  F
           b.  T
           c.  T
           d.  T
           e.  T

The virus is readily inactivated by heat and by sodium hypochlorite.

**Q.10.6   A positive blood test indicates that the patient:**

a. Has AIDS
b. Has been exposed to HIV virus
c. Has persistent infection
d. Can transmit the virus
e. Has natural immunity to AIDS

**Q.10.7   Early AIDS may present with:**

a. A seroconversion illness like glandular fever
b. Arthralgia
c. Perianal herpes simplex
d. Retrosternal discomfort and dysphagia
e. Acute encephalopathy

**Q.10.8   Acute encephalopathy may present as:**

a. Loss of memory
b. Slowness of thought
c. Loss of balance
d. Difficulty in pronunciation
e. Personality change

**Q.10.9   AIDS patients may have:**

a. Intermittent fever
b. Weight loss
c. Extreme malaise
d. Night sweats
e. Diarrhoea

**Q.10.10 Patients with established AIDS may present with:**

a. Lymphadenopathy
b. Hairy leukoplakia
c. Pneumonia
d. Kaposi's sarcoma
e. Lymphoma of the anorectum

**For answers see over**

# Answers

**A.10.6**  a. F
       b. T
       c. T
       d. T
       e. F

**A.10.7**  a. T
       b. T
       c. T
       d. T
       e. T

**A.10.8**  a. T
       b. T
       c. T
       d. T
       e. T

Acute encepalopathy may proceed to dementia.

**A.10.9**  a. T
       b. T
       c. T
       d. T
       e. T

Differential diagnosis includes active tuberculosis, *Cryptococcus* infection and colitis. AIDS compounds the risk of acquiring tuberculosis.

**A.10.10**  a. T
        b. T
        c. T
        d. T
        e. T

Lesions of the mouth, anus or rectum may be a non-Hodgkin's lymphoma or a squamous cell carcinoma.

**Q.10.11  Advanced AIDS patients have:**

    a. Foxy facial features
    b. Coarse voices
    c. Slow speech
    d. Difficulty in pronunciation
    e. Dementia

**Q.10.12  Meningitis in AIDS is confirmed by:**

    a. Computed tomography
    b. Electroencephalography
    c. Culture of the cerebrospinal fluid
    d. Cryptococcal antigen in serum
    e. Cryptococcal antigen in the cerebrospinal fluid

**Q.10.13  *Pneumocystis carinii* pneumonia:**

    a. Is protozoal infection
    b. Affects alveolar spaces
    c. Is life-threatening in AIDS
    d. Is characterised by a productive cough
    e. Is best treated with co-trimoxazole, trimethoprim and sulphamethoxazole

**Q.10.14  The high-risk groups for AIDS include:**

    a. Men who have had anal intercourse with other men since 1977
    b. Drug abusers who have injected themselves and shared needles in the past 10 years
    c. Haemophiliacs who have received blood products within the last 5–10 years
    d. People who have lived in or visited Central Africa at any time since 1977 and have had sex with men or women there
    e. Bisexuals

**For answers see over**

**A.10.11** a. T
b. T
c. T
d. T
e. T

**A.10.12** a. F
b. F
c. T
d. T
e. T

The meningitis is due to the fungus *Cryptococcus neoformans*.

**A.10.13** a. T
b. T
c. T
d. F
e. T

**A.10.14** a. T
b. T
c. T
d. T
e. T

# 11.  *Hepatitis B*

**Q.11.1  Hepatitis B may be transmitted by:**

    a.  Shared needles in drug addicts
    b.  Contaminated food
    c.  Airborne droplet infection
    d.  Shared razors
    e.  Needle sticks

**Q.11.2  Hepatitis B:**

    a.  Can be prevented by immunisation
    b.  Confers immunity on those infected
    c.  Has an incubation period of 30 days
    d.  Can be fatal
    e.  May be transmitted by AIDS sufferers

**Q.11.3  The following high-risk groups should be screened for hepatitis B:**

    a.  Tattooed patients
    b.  Haemophiliacs
    c.  The elderly in institutions
    d.  The mentally handicapped in institutions
    e.  Blood donors

**Q.11.4  In the UK serological evidence of exposure to hepatitis B virus is:**

    a.  0–2% of the normal population
    b.  2%–5% of the normal population
    c.  5%–10% of the normal population
    d.  10%–15% of the normal population
    e.  15%–20% of the normal population

**Q.11.5  The incidence of infection amongst hospital medical staff is:**

    a.  0–5 per 100 000
    b.  5–10 per 100 000
    c.  10–30 per 100 000
    d.  30–50 per 100 000
    e.  50–70 per 100 000

**For answers see over**

**A.11.1**  a.  T
          b.  F
          c.  F
          d.  T
          e.  T

**A.11.2**  a.  T
          b.  T
          c.  F
          d.  T
          e.  T

The incubation period of hepatitis B is 6 weeks to 3 months.

It is fatal in 2%–3% of cases.

**A.11.3**  a.  T
          b.  T
          c.  F
          d.  T
          e.  F

**A.11.4**  a.  F
          b.  T
          c.  F
          d.  F
          e.  F

**A.11.5**  a.  F
          b.  F
          c.  T
          d.  F
          e.  F

**Q.11.6   The high-risk medical staff are in:**

    a.  Pathology performing necropsies
    b.  Accident and Emergency Department
    c.  Theatre
    d.  Renal unit
    e.  Genitourinary unit

**Q.11.7   Spillage of blood or body fluid should be:**

    a.  Mopped or wiped with bleach
    b.  Treated with Virusorb powder
    c.  Wiped with methylated spirit
    d.  Wiped with povidone iodine
    e.  Washed with hot water and detergent

**Q.11.8   With needle stick injuries:**

    a.  Wash thoroughly
    b.  Encourage bleeding
    c.  Report to senior medical staff
    d.  Establish the hepatitis B antigen status of the patient
    e.  Give tetanus toxoid booster

**For answers see over**

# Answers

**A.11.6**  a.  T
       b.  T
       c.  T
       d.  T
       e.  T

**A.11.7**  a.  T
       b.  T
       c.  F
       d.  F
       e.  T

Spillage should be mopped or wiped (wearing gloves) after treating with bleach 1 part in 10 parts water.

An alternative way is to apply Virusorb powder, which contains chloramine T, to the spillage and allow to set. It can then be scooped up and disposed of. Either method destroys the human immunodeficiency virus (HIV) and the hepatitis B virus (HBV).

Instruments may be decontaminated by soaking in freshly prepared glutaraldehyde 2% for 1 hour, washing with detergent and soaking again in glutaraldehyde for 3 hours.

Contaminated bed linen may be put in a washing machine. Ten minutes at 90 °C is adequate to inactivate the virus.

**A.11.8**  a.  T
       b.  T
       c.  T
       d.  T
       e.  T

Watch what you stick where, with what and with whom.

Wear gloves when taking blood and putting in cannulae.

Wear gloves when dealing with bleeding.

Don't cap the needle, discard it in the Sharps box.

Over 40% of needle sticks are due to re-sheathing the needle.

When performing gastric lavage it is advisable to wear eye protection, mask and plastic apron.

Think HIV positive and think HBV positive.

# 12. *Pot-pourri*

**Q.12.1 Superglue contamination:**

    a. Of the eyelids should be treated by irrigation with warm saline or water and the eye covered with a pad for 24 hours

    b. Of the fingers may be managed by application of nitromethane

    c. Of the fingers may be managed by separating the fingers

    d. Of the lips may be managed by bathing in warm soapy water

    e. Of the lips may be managed by forcing apart the lips

**Q.12.2 In the management of dog and cat bites:**

    a. The treatment is the same

    b. Both require tetanus toxoid

    c. Penicillin is routinely administered

    d. Sepsis is unlikely

    e. Any infection is Gram-positive

**Q.12.3 After drinking 5 measures of whisky or 2½ pints of beer the blood alcohol level after 75 minutes will be:**

    a. 40 mg

    b. 50 mg

    c. 60 mg

    d. 70 mg

    e. 90 mg

**For answers see over**

# Answers

**A.12.1**  a. T
          b. T
          c. F
          d. T
          e. F

Superglue is a cyanocrylate adhesive and may bond skin in seconds. Immersing the affected part in warm soapy water may be followed by application of nitromethane if unsuccessful. Nitromethane should not be used for the eyes.

The patient is sometimes the victim of a practical joker and may be brought to the accident department attached to an object such as a ladder or a toilet seat.

**A.12.2**  a. F
          b. T
          c. F
          d. F
          e. F

Dog bites generally heal without infection. Cat bites often become severely infected; the bacterium is *Pasteurella,* which is sensitive to amoxicillin and co-trimoxazole. The treatment of choice for cat bites is co-trimoxazole with metronidazole.

**A.12.3**  a. F
          b. F
          c. F
          d. F
          e. T

**Q.12.4** **The degradation rate of alcohol is:**

a. 5 mg per 100 ml per hour
b. 10 mg per 100 ml per hour
c. 15 mg per 100 ml per hour
d. 20 mg per 100 ml per hour
e. 25 mg per 100 ml per hour

**Q.12.5** **Athetoid movements and acute dyskinesia:**

a. May present as torticollis
b. May be extrapyramidal
c. May result from phenothiazine
d. May follow vomiting treated with metoclopramide
e. May be abolished by IV benztropine

**For answers see over**

# Answers

**A.12.4**  a. F
b. F
c. T
d. F
e. F

It thus takes 6 hours to remove alcohol from the blood after 5 whiskies or 2½ pints of beer.

Alcometer readings are useful in an Accident and Emergency Department. If the level is below 300 mg in an unconscious patient the unconsciousness is unlikely to be due to alcohol.

An unresponsive patient smelling of alcohol should have a skull X-ray.

500 ml 20% laevulose, 100 g IV, will increase the degradation rate of alcohol by 20–30 mg per 100 ml in 1 hour.

---

**Alcohol and Road Traffic Accidents**

Thirty-three per cent of drivers involved in road traffic accidents (RTAs) between 6 p.m. and midnight have blood alcohol levels of between 50 and 100 mg. After midnight 50% of drivers have blood alcohol levels of over 50 mg and 33% have levels over 100 mg.

Fifty per cent of pedestrians involved in RTAs between 6 p.m. and midnight have blood alcohol levels of over 50 mg and 33% have levels over 100 mg. After midnight almost 100% of pedestrians involved in RTAs have blood alcohol levels over 100 mg.

---

**A.12.5**  a. T
b. T
c. T
d. T
e. T

The response to 1 mg benztropine intravenously in drug-induced acute dyskinesia is dramatic and perhaps the quickest cure in the emergency room.

### Q.12.6  In torticollis:

a. There is spasm of one sternomastoid muscle
b. The head is turned to the opposite side
c. The onset is often spontaneous
d. Flexion and extension are possible
e. A submandibular abscess must be excluded

### Q.12.7  Hyperkinesia in children may be due to:

a. Food additives
b. Antibiotic suspension
c. Threadworms
d. Hyperthyroidism
e. Amphetamines

### Q.12.8  A membrane of the throat which bleeds on swabbing is due to:

a. Tonsillitis
b. Vincent's angina
c. Diphtheria
d. Glandular fever
e. Quinsy

### Q.12.9  Dysphagia may be due to:

a. Pharyngitis
b. Foreign body
c. Pseudobulbar palsy
d. Malignancy
c. Herpes virus

### Q.12.10  Quinsy:

a. Commonly affects young people
b. Is a retropharyngeal abscess
c. Is characterised by dysphagia and salivation
d. Causes displacement of the uvula
e. Requires general anaesthetic for incision

**For answers see over**

# Answers

**A.12.6**  a. T
        b. F
        c. T
        d. T
        e. T

The head is turned to the affected side.

**A.12.7**  a. T
        b. T
        c. F
        d. T
        e. T

Tartrazine (E102) is a common additive to food and antibiotic suspensions that can cause hyperkinesia.

**A.12.8**  a. F
        b. F
        c. T
        d. F
        e. F

**A.12.9**  a. T
        b. T
        c. T
        d. T
        e. T

Herpes virus ulceration of the throat or pharynx may be an early presentation in AIDS.

**A.12.10**  a. F
        b. F
        c. T
        d. T
        e. F

Quinsy is a peritonsillar abscess.

### Q.12.11 Acute oedema of the glottis:

a. May be due to anaphylaxis
b. Is characterised by dysphagia
c. May be due to corrosive fluids
d. Has the appearance of a cervix on laryngoscopy
e. Affects the vocal cords

### Q.12.12 Choking and inhalation of a foreign body:

a. Should be treated by patting the back
b. Should be treated from behind by applying sudden thrusts below the xiphisternum
c. Should be treated by turning the patient upside down
d. May be due to food, sweets or peanuts
e. Via the trachea goes down the left bronchus

### Q.12.13 Otitic barotrauma:

a. Affects the middle ear
b. Is due to positive pressure
c. Occurs in descent in flying
d. Occurs in diving and underwater descent
e. May occur in a hyperbaric chamber

**For answers see over**

# Answers

**A.12.11**  a. T
        b. T
        c. T
        d. T
        e. F

**A.12.12**  a. F
        b. T
        c. F
        d. T
        e. F

The manoeuvre from behind is known as the Heimlich manoeuvre, described by Dr. Henry Heimlich of Cincinatti in 1974. The rescuer joins his hands over his wrist below the victim's xiphisternum and produces sudden repeated bear-hugs. If this is unsuccessful laryngoscopy and/or bronchoscopy is performed.

An inhaled peanut – often resulting from throwing one into the air and attempting to catch it in the mouth – goes down the right bronchus.

**A.12.13**  a. T
        b. F
        c. T
        d. T
        e. T

Otitic barotrauma is due to negative pressure relative to the environment and occurs most often during air travel.

**Q.12.14  Vertigo:**

    a. Occurs in Ménière's disease
    b. Occurs in vestibular neuronitis
    c. May be positional
    d. May occur in cervical spondylosis
    e. Occurs in acute labyrinthitis secondary to middle ear disease

**Q.12.15  Hiccup:**

    a. Is often due to gastric distention
    b. Is common in hiatus hernia
    c. Occurs in uraemia
    d. If persistent, necessitates chest X-ray
    e. May be treated with chlorpromazine IM

**Q.12.16  Foreign bodies in the stomach:**

    a. Should have routine gastroscopy
    b. Should always be removed
    c. If multiple have been swallowed intentionally
    d. Can always be seen on X-ray
    e. Usually impact in the ileum

**Q.12.17  Recent epigastric pain in an elderly man is likely to be due to:**

    a. Angina
    b. Peptic ulcer
    c. Oesophageal regurgitation
    d. Pancreatitis
    e. Alcohol

**For answers see over**

# Answers

**A.12.14**  a.  T
            b.  T
            c.  T
            d.  T
            e.  T

In Ménière's disease there is usually deafness and tinnitus. As the deafness increases the vertigo often settles. The disease is uncommon before middle age.

Sudden onset of vertigo without deafness following an upper respiratory infection is suggestive of vestibular neuronitis.

Benign positional vertigo is fairly common.

In cervical spondylosis there may be compression of the vertebral artery on movement of the neck resulting in brainstem ischaemia. A bruit may be heard over the carotid or vertebral artery.

Chronic ear infection causing labyrinthitis is obvious from the history and clinical examination.

**A.12.15**  a.  T
            b.  F
            c.  T
            d.  T
            e.  T

A chest X-ray is advisable in persistent hiccup to exclude subphrenic abscess.

**A.12.16**  a.  F
            b.  F
            c.  T
            d.  F
            e.  F

**A.12.17**  a.  F
            b.  F
            c.  T
            d.  T
            e.  T

**Q.12.18  Acute pancreatitis:**

    a.  Is characterised by acute epigastric pain radiating to the back
    b.  May be associated with gall stones
    c.  Has abdominal rigidity occurring early in the attack
    d.  Commonly produces lilac discoloration of the skin of the upper abdomen
    e.  Produces serum amylase peaks at 48 hours

**Q.12.19  Ureteric colic:**

    a.  Is acute pain radiating from loin to groin
    b.  Is associated with pyrexia
    c.  Is characterised by rigidity of the rectus abdominis
    d.  Is usually associated with a tender palpable kidney
    e.  Always produces haematuria

**For answers see over**

# Answers

**A.12.18**   a. T
b. T
c. F
d. F
e. F

Rigidity of the abdominal wall occurs 3–4 hours after the onset. The abdomen is usually soft in the initial stage of shock.

Discoloration of the skin is not a common manifestation but may arise 2 or 3 days later; it is seen in the loins where transversalis to the spinae joins.

Serum amylase levels are maximum between 2 and 12 hours and return to normal between 48 and 72 hours after the acute episode.

**A.12.19**   a. T
b. F
c. F
d. F
e. F

The temperature is usually subnormal.

The lateral abdominal muscles are rigid but not the rectus abdominis.

The kidney is palpable only if the calculus causes hydronephrosis or pyonephrosis.

Haematuria occurs in 50% cases; the urine is often smoky in appearance.

The Munchausen patient often presents in an Accident and Emergency Department simulating ureteric colic to obtain pethidine. He/she knows the characteristic radiation of pain and can produce sweating and vomiting. A sample of urine may contain fresh blood from a self-induced finger prick.

**Q.12.20 Haematemesis in cirrhosis:**

    a. Is due to rupture of oesophageal varices
    b. Is painful
    c. Is treated with a Sengstaken tube
    d. Is treated with vasopressin
    e. Is treated by thoracotomy

**Q.12.21 Charcot's biliary triad includes:**

    a. Recurrent pain
    b. Pruritus
    c. Fluctuating jaundice
    d. Pale stools
    e. Fever and rigors

**Q.12.22 Raynaud's syndrome:**

    a. Affects the peripheral limb arteries
    b. Has an attributable cause
    c. May be due to cervical rib
    d. May be associated with ergot poisoning
    e. May result from the use of pneumatic drills

**Q.12.23 Raynaud's disease:**

    a. Is bilateral
    b. Is excessive vessel reaction to cold
    c. Is characterised by cold dead fingers with pain and paraesthesia
    d. Is equally common in men and women
    e. Is part of generalised organic vascular disease

**For answers see over**

# Answers

A.12.20    a.   T
           b.   F
           c.   T
           d.   T
           e.   T

Painless haematemesis is often severe and massive and the cause of death if the bleeding is not arrested. Urgent blood transfusion is indicated.

A Sengstaken triple lumen tube is passed. The gastric balloon is inflated at the oesophago-gastric junction. The oesophageal balloon is inflated in the lower oesophagus at a pressure of 25 mmHg. The stomach contents are aspirated hourly. The oesophageal balloon is deflated every 24 hours to avoid oesophageal ulceration. A ruptured ulcer may cause fatal mediastinitis. Neomycin is introduced down the gastric tube.

Freshly prepared vasopressin, 20 units of 5%, is given intravenously in 20 minutes to reduce portal pressure.

If bleeding is not controlled the patient is referred for surgery.

A.12.21    a.   T
           b.   F
           c.   T
           d.   F
           e.   T

A.12.22    a.   T
           b.   T
           c.   T
           d.   T
           e.   T

A.12.23    a.   T
           b.   T
           c.   T
           d.   F
           e.   F

Raynaud's disease is more common in women.

### Q.12.24 Thrombophlebitis:

a. May follow trauma
b. Is characterised by pain and tenderness
c. May produce embolism
d. Requires support and analgesia
e. Requires anticoagulant treatment

### Q.12.25 Deep vein thrombosis:

a. May occur after surgery
b. Commonly develops in the soleus muscle of the calf
c. May embolise
d. Produces a positive Homans' sign
e. Causes oedema of the ankle

### Q.12.26 Acute pain in the face:

a. May be trigeminal neuralgia
b. May be associated with endogenous depression
c. May be migrainous
d. May be due to herpes zoster
e. May arise from an aneurysm within the cavernous sinus

**For answers see over**

# Answers

**A.12.24**   a.  T
         b.  T
         c.  F
         d.  T
         e.  F

In thrombophlebitis the clot is firmly attached to an inflamed intima, progresses to fibrosis and organisation and there may be recanalisation of the vein. Embolism rarely occurs. Anticoagulants are not indicated.

**A.12.25**   a.  T
         b.  T
         c.  T
         d.  T
         e.  F

Deep vein thrombosis is due to stasis. The clot is friable and loosely attached to the intima and may become detached resulting in pulmonary embolism. The majority of thromboses occur in the large venous sinuses of the soleus muscle of the calf.

Pain in the calf produced by passively dorsiflexing the foot is Homans' sign. There is marked tenderness of the lower soleus muscle.

Oedema of the ankle does not appear unless the thrombus extends to the popliteal vein obstructing venous return.

Diagnosis is confirmed by intravenous $^{125}$I-fibrinogen.

Heparin may be administered prior to surgery and afterwards as a prophylactic measure.

The treatment of deep vein thrombosis is by the administration of anticoagulants or thrombectomy.

**A.12.26**   a.  T
         b.  T
         c.  T
         d.  T
         e.  T

Many psychiatric patients complain of symptoms more suggestive of organic than mental disease. Facial pain may be the presenting somatic complaint in endogenous depression.

**Q.12.27 Respiratory distress may be due to:**

    a. Acute left ventricular failure
    b. Acute asthma
    c. Smoke inhalation
    d. Inhaled foreign body
    e. Stridor

**Q.12.28 In acute left ventricular failure:**

    a. Morphine is indicated
    b. Diuretics should be given IM
    c. Oxygen is of value
    d. The patient is managed sitting head up
    e. Aggravating factors – dysrhythmias, anaemia and hypertension – should be corrected

**Q.12.29 Chest pain may be due to:**

    a. Acute myocardial infarction
    b. Angina
    c. Pneumothorax
    d. Oesophagitis
    e. Bornholm disease

**Q.12.30 Bornholm disease:**

    a. Is characterised by severe chest pain on inspiration
    b. Is also known as epidemic pleurodynia
    c. Is due to coxsackie B virus
    d. May be complicated by orchitis
    e. Is afebrile

**For answers see over**

# Answers

**A.12.27**  a.  T
           b.  T
           c.  T
           d.  T
           e.  T

**A.12.28**  a.  T
           b.  F
           c.  T
           d.  T
           e.  T

Acute left ventricular failure and pulmonary oedema usually respond well to morphine and frusemide IV. Failure to respond is an indication for pulmonary artery pressure monitoring with a Swan–Ganz catheter.

**A.12.29**  a.  T
           b.  T
           c.  T
           d.  T
           e.  T

**A.12.30**  a.  T
           b.  T
           c.  T
           d.  T
           e.  F

Bornholm disease, or Devil's grip, has been known for a hundred years but is often forgotten as a cause of acute chest pain. Bornholm is a Scandinavian island under the Danish flag. The disease is associated with fever and is self-limiting.

**Q.12.31  Ventricular tachycardia:**

    a. Is best treated with intravenous lignocaine following myocardial infarction
    b. May be treated with DC shock
    c. May be treated with verapamil
    d. May be treated with beta-blockers
    e. May be treated with flecainide

**Q.12.32  Beta-adrenoceptor blockers:**

    a. Are used in the treatment of hypertension
    b. Reduce the recurrence rate of myocardial infarction
    c. Are used in heart failure
    d. Improve exercise tolerance in angina
    e. May precipitate asthma

**Q.12.33  Acute pulmonary embolism may be associated with:**

    a. Syncope
    b. Low arterial $pO_2$
    c. High arterial $pCO_2$
    d. Normal perfusion scan
    e. An ECG showing left ventricular strain

**Q.12.34  Legionnaires' disease:**

    a. Is pneumonia caused by *Legionella pneumophila*
    b. Occurs in epidemics
    c. Arises from shower units, air conditioning and cooling towers
    d. Affects young people
    e. Affects non-smokers

**For answers see over**

# Answers

**A.12.31**  a.  T
            b.  T
            c.  F
            d.  F
            e.  T

Verapamil (5 mg slowly IV) is used in the treatment of supraventricular tachycardia.

Beta-blockers may be used to control supraventricular tachycardia following myocardial infarction. Practolol 5 mg should be given IV.

**A.12.32**  a.  T
            b.  T
            c.  F
            d.  T
            e.  T

**A.12.33**  a.  T
            b.  T
            c.  F
            d.  F
            e.  F

The arterial $pCO_2$ is low.

The perfusion scan is abnormal.

The ECG shows right ventricular strain and often S1 Q3 T3.

**A.12.34**  a.  T
            b.  T
            c.  T
            d.  F
            e.  F

Legionnaires' disease affects men more than women, in the mid-50s age group.

It affects heavy smokers and drinkers.

It is more common in summer than winter.

The incubation period is 2–10 days.

**Q.12.35  Legionnaires' disease is characterised by:**

    a.  Malaise and headache
    b.  Myalgia and arthralgia
    c.  Fever
    d.  Tachycardia
    e.  Cough and haemoptysis

**Q.12.36  Confusional states may be related to:**

    a.  Alcohol intoxication or withdrawal
    b.  Hypoglycaemia
    c.  Myxoedema
    d.  Anaemia
    e.  Psychoses and dementia

**Q.12.37  Hypopituitarism:**

    a.  Is due to destruction of the posterior lobe of the pituitary gland
    b.  Results from postpartum haemorrhage
    c.  Is characterised by failure of lactation and amenorrhoea
    d.  Is characterised by absent or scanty pubic hair
    e.  Is characterised by secondary hypothyroidism and hypo-adrenalism

**Q.12.38  Tietze syndrome is:**

    a.  Epidemic myalgia
    b.  Tuberculosis of a rib
    c.  A painful swelling of the second or third costal cartilage
    d.  Common in elderly men
    e.  Treated by irradiation

**For answers see over**

# Answers

**A.12.35**  a.  T
        b.  T
        c.  T
        d.  F
        e.  T

The temperature may be > 40 °C and there is a relative brady-cardia.

The treatment is erythromycin 500 mg q.d.s. for 3 weeks.

**A.12.36**  a.  T
        b.  T
        c.  T
        d.  T
        e.  T

An elderly patient may be clinically disturbed as a result of anaemia due to vitamin $B_{12}$ deficiency.

**A.12.37**  a.  F
        b.  T
        c.  T
        d.  T
        e.  T

Hypopituitarism results from infarction of the anterior lobe of the pituitary gland following postpartum haemorrhage.

The diagnosis may be confused with anorexia nervosa.

In anorexia nervosa there is gross wasting, no appetite and normal distribution of pubic hair. In anorexia the response to corticosteroids is poor, but is good in hypopituitarism.

**A.12.38**  a.  F
        b.  F
        c.  T
        d.  F
        e.  F

Tietze syndrome affects both sexes in the third or fourth decade. The aetiology is unknown and the disorder is self-limiting.

**Q.12.39  Triage:**

     a.  Means "separation"
     b.  Is from the French word *"tirer"*
     c.  Means "a threesome"
     d.  Refers to coffee beans
     e.  Means "to try"

**For answers see over**

# Answers

**A.12.39**  a.  T
        b.  F
        c.  F
        d.  T
        e.  F

The word triage refers to the separation of broken and whole coffee beans. It is derived from the French *"trier"*, meaning to sort. In recent times it has become associated with the sorting of the injured and acutely ill. A triage nurse is stationed at the reception of many major Accident and Emergency Departments in the UK and emergency rooms in the United States. Forms of triage, however, were carried out by the Ancient Greeks, the Romans, and in the nineteenth century by Baron Larrey, Napoleon's surgeon.